Big Girls Do It Running:

Health, Fitness, and Kicking Life's Ass!

My journey from 430lbs to fit AND fabulous

Jasinda Wilder

Praise for Big Girls Do It Running

You have nothing to lose but weight, right? What better way to learn than with someone who has been through the trenches, put in the work, done the research, and has found a solution that works? I believe in Jasinda as a friend, an author, and now as a pioneer. You will too! — *Pamela C, 37*

This was the simplest change I could ever make. It was super easy to do and I really didn't have to think about it at all. All you do is eat, walk or jog, and you lose weight. It couldn't be simpler than that. — *Jennifer O, 34*

One of my favorite things to come from this experience is that my whole family has become involved. We're in the kitchen together most nights cooking dinners, and we eat out a lot less. But I love that it is not difficult at all to stay within our lifestyle changes on evenings when we do choose to eat out. I don't feel deprived; I can still have chocolate and ice cream. I don't have to weigh out perfect portions; I don't have to leave the table hungry or unsatisfied, and there is no calorie counting. There are none of the things in this program that made me give up on past attempts at weight loss. —*Andrea G, 40*

The *Big Girls Do It Running* revolution has truly saved me. At the start of this year I was frustrated and didn't know where to turn, or what other diet I could possibly try. This process is has been so successful for me because Jasinda herself has experienced the same struggles so many of us have. Thank you, Jasinda, for being such a light to in my life. I am so grateful for you and your guidance. I feel my life is being transformed. I feel I am discovering my true self! Thank you from the bottom of my heart! — *Donna K, 38*

This woman and her program have saved my life. A few weeks before being selected for this wonderful journey I was told I was going blind because of my diabetes. My blood sugars have always run in the 300s, even with up to six insulin injections a day. At this point I had given up in on life. This program has gotten got me off insulin in four weeks. For the first time in 15 years my blood sugar is normal. Jasinda has helped me to be able to see for many years to come. — *Sara W, 28*

As a single girl living in a big city, it's important that I can eat meals out, and this plan not only lets me do that, but it makes it easy to do! *The Wilder Way* does take some adjustment, but once you get used to it, it feels natural and easy. It's something you can live with for the rest of your life and never feel deprived. I will always be grateful to Jasinda for inviting me to be part of this process and for helping me change my health and my body for the better. — *Michelle K, 32*

Jasinda Wilder's plan, *The Wilder Way,* is educational and easy to follow. You don't have to count calories or measure out everything you eat. There are no bland, prepackaged meals, no chalky shakes to choke down, no starving yourself; you eat *REAL* food. Not only does *The Wilder Way* provide you with delicious new recipes to try, but also healthier versions of old favorites like cookies and cake! This is not a diet, fad, or gimmick, it's a plan you will want to continue for life. I have accomplished some amazing things in just eight weeks: I've lost pounds and inches, I've gone from a sedentary lifestyle to participating in a 5K, I've kicked my pop habit...and I've been able to stop taking one of my daily medications. Most importantly, I feel better, physically and mentally, than I have in YEARS. — *Kerry G, 44*

Foreword

First, let me thank you for picking up this book. I hope if you or someone you know are struggling with the same issues I have struggled with, namely maintaining a healthy weight and lifestyle, that *BIG GIRLS DO IT RUNNING* will offer insights and encouragement to help you move forward.

But, before you begin reading, I want you to know that I am *not* a health expert. In fact, I'm about the farthest thing from an expert you could imagine. I'm just a mom, a wife, and a daughter with a little bit of wisdom and a lot of personal experience to share. I truly hope that by sharing my journey I will be able to help anyone who is trying to look at their health and their life in a different way.

This book is written from my personal perspective only, and the information contained herein should by no means be considered a substitute for the advice of a qualified medical professional.

Always consult your physician before beginning any new exercise or health program. Every effort has been made to ensure the accuracy of the information contained in this book as of the date of publication. The author and publisher (that's me!) expressly disclaim responsibility for any adverse effects arising from the use, or application, of the information contained herein.

Jasinda Wilder
February 2016

Dedication

First, this book is dedicated to my husband, who sees me as beautiful on my best days as well as my worst: I couldn't do this life without you. TODAAT-CWM

Second, this book is for my children who inspire me every single day to be the best I can be. You are my heart and soul. Don't forget to beast mode at the end—you won't regret it. I'm so proud of you!

And finally, this book is for my parents, who always tried so hard to help me find health; I've finally found it. Thank you for never giving up on me and pushing me to always be my best. I wouldn't be who I am today without your love and guidance.

Acknowledgements

This book would not have been possible without the support from so many special people in my life.

Thank you to my dear friends Karri and Meredith, who fill in all the gaps in my life and our crazy schedule, from testing recipes to picking up the slack around the house and folding laundry. You ladies are the best. Thank you from the bottom of my heart.

To my amazing photographer Leah, and my graphic designer Sarah: Thank you so much for working so hard to give this book a special look and feel. You drip talent and I'm so grateful to be able to work with you both.

To my editor Valerie, who didn't balk when I told her I wanted to do a non-fiction project: thank you for believing in me and in this body of work. You are invaluable in our writing process. Thank you!

To my agent Kristin Nelson, who is always willing to help me with my indie projects when she gets paid almost nothing to do so. Thank you! Your support and constant help and guidance with this project has been nothing short of amazing. The team at Nelson Literary Agency is simply the best of the best.

And last but certainly not least, I would like to extend a special and heartfelt thank you to the twenty-five brave, beautiful, and kick-ass warrior women who volunteered to be my beta test group for The Wilder Way. You amaze me, and you inspire me. Thank you so much for trusting me with eight weeks of your lives, and for taking this incredible step toward health with me. Let's start a revolution, ladies!

Contents

PART 1:

My Backstory

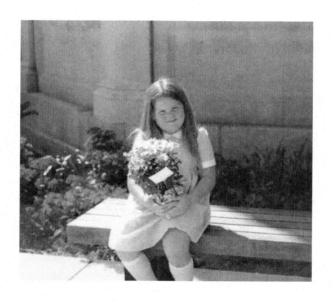

Chapter 1

BEING A FAT KID SUCKS

"*TWO THINGS GET ME IN TROUBLE: FOOD AND MY MOUTH*". IF you've read my best-selling fiction series *Big Girls Do It,* then you're familiar with that opening line. What you may not know is that those books are partially autobiographical.

Before I wrote that series I'd read several romances and erotic romances and found myself struggling to identify with the female leads. They just…weren't people I could identify with. For one thing, they were all described as being thin and svelte, images of the way Hollywood and the marketing industry depicts the epitome of female beauty and perfection. And ladies…that ain't me. Never has been, and never will be. So I wrote *Big Girls Do It Better* in an attempt to write a story featuring a hot, sexy, self-confident female lead that also happened to be 'not skinny'. My heroine was a big girl, and she rocked it. Like just about every woman out there, she also had her self-doubts, her hang-ups and insecurities, but she didn't let them keep her down, and she didn't let them stop her from going after what—and whom—she wanted.

Now, if it were my mother telling this story she would say I weighed close to a hundred pounds at one year of age, and that she was always worried about my size. But then, she also swears that I'm a MENSA level genius, so she probably shouldn't be trusted too far.

No, I didn't weigh quite *that* much at that age, but it is true that my weight is something I've always struggled with. But, the truth is, I can't really remember the first time I realized I was fat. What I actually remember more is thinking that something was wrong with me. It all started when I was around four or five years old—as I was getting ready to start school—and my mom told me I needed to go to the hospital for some "genetic testing." I wasn't really sure what that meant, exactly, but I was certainly aware that I'd been crowned the tallest four year-old in the state of Michigan—you can check it out, I'm in the medical books.

Our pediatrician told my mother that he was concerned I might be an actual, literal giant. At that age, one of my favorite things to watch on TV was wrestling. The only giant I knew was Andre the Giant, and I *really* didn't want to end up looking like him. At that age I couldn't even comprehend what actually having gigantism might mean for me, or what medical problems I might have as a result of it. All I knew was that I just didn't want it.

So I was taken to the hospital and they started doing tests on my growth. I was there for days, and they took vial after vial of my blood. After endless batteries of tests were completed, and I was poked and prodded until I felt like an alien abductee or some kind of medical experiment, we were told that they could find nothing wrong with me, I was just going to be a big girl, with big feet, big hands, a big head, and—as I would later discover—a really, *really* big booty.

Having a big booty wasn't a big deal when I was five years old, but as I continued to grow, so did my health problems. I developed asthma so severe I couldn't run or dance for very long without needing an inhaler. Despite my physical issues, I continued to be a very active child. I danced, swam, played basketball, and softball.

But the real problem wasn't too much physical activity, it was food.

See, fat kids like cake. *All* kids like cake—okay, okay, *most* kids like cake, unless they're weird, in which case they probably prefer carrots or something. I was raised in an era when most birthday parties happened at McDonalds, when you tried all thirty-one flavors at Baskin-Robbins, and ate pizza at least once a week. As far as I was concerned, growing up in suburban Detroit was pretty great.

Then the pediatrician decided it would be best to shift our efforts and consult a pediatric nutritionist. What this meant was that I started going to Weight Watchers® with my mother.

And this is when things really took a turn for the worse.

Back in the 80s everyone was afraid of being overweight, and they were afraid of anything to do with the word *FAT*—that word represented everything that was big, bad and evil in our society. Anything that contained "fats" was taboo. Fats were declared to be the enemy. Real butter. Cheese. Cream. Nuts. Oils in food. These are all fats, and these were said to be the problem. Fats make you fat, right? That was the thinking of the day but, happily, we now know better.

I remember my nutritionist giving my mother and me a list of "free foods"—these were foods I could eat at any time, and I could have as much of them as I wanted. These foods were "free" because they were all "fat free." I distinctly remember angel food cake being one of the "free foods" on the list. I didn't even really *like* angel food cake, but since it was cake, and since I could eat as much as I wanted, I took full advantage. Meaning, I ate about half a cake per day. Free cake? Hell, yeah! And even though I was only in elementary school, I remember thinking this was really weird. How could *cake* be fat free, and be good for me at the same time?

During that period my weight kept going up and my nutrition-ist was baffled. I was eating exactly what she had told me to eat; yet I wasn't losing any weight. When I noticed my weight wasn't going down, I started sneaking foods that were not on my approved list be-cause what was the point? Why just eat shitty cake all day if I wasn't going to lose any weight?

I think the most weight I lost in the two years we attended those Weight Watcher® meetings was maybe five pounds. My mom stocked our fridge full of frozen diet meals and desserts, but if the package came with two portions, I would eat both. Why not? I mean, if you're ten years old and both Weight Watchers® *and* a nutritionist can't help you lose weight then why not eat two full meals and half an angel food cake every day? After all, it's diet food!

As you can see, my health and my mindset were both going straight down hill, *fast.* I think I gained about a hundred pounds during elementary school. The strange thing was, however, that even though my body was on a downward spiral, other things seemed to be okay. I was pretty funny, I had friends, I continued to dance and sing. Sure, I was the butt of some jokes, because not everyone could deal with me being 5'8" in 4th grade, or wearing women's size 11 shoes. I remember hearing people yelling out how much they guessed I'd weigh by sixth grade. I was well aware of the cruelty of it, keenly so, but I was also aware that everyone had some sort of trau-ma to overcome. To boost my confidence, I told myself I was going to rock this body, whether everyone was on board or not…

And then I'd secretly eat an entire box of Pop Tarts in my room after I got home from school.

One of my most vivid memories from sixth grade was being beaten up during recess by several of the boys in my class. Did they think that because I was the biggest kid in my class it would be cool to take me on? I don't know, maybe they were all secretly hot for me? Yeah, let's just go with that. So, as if it wasn't bad enough getting thrown to the ground and having the shit kicked out of me by seven of the "cool guys", it was even more humiliating when someone told the principal what had happened. The result was that all seven of those cool kids had to personally apologize to me. God, that was awful. Now they all hated me, *and* they thought I had tattled on them to the principal. Later that day I was followed home from school by two of the boys who threw rocks at me the whole way. I'd officially been labeled a freak.

That event marked the first but, sadly, not the last time a boy would hit me—but more on that later.

In his goodness, God threw me a break even as I was experiencing these new terrible feelings about myself. I had a decent group of friends and I was getting positive attention for my singing voice, so I kept myself busy with singing and music.

Privately, however, my self-esteem was pretty much in the gutter. I'd had a few innocent pre-pubescent crushes but, overall, boys were just scary to me. Food was my coping mechanism. I ate away my problems and that helped to keep most of the bad emotions at bay. I made a fortress around myself with Twinkies and Ding Dongs and Pop Tarts.

Now, I'm not saying I didn't eat healthy stuff too; I never had any issues with vegetables, fish, or salads—I would eat almost anything. But my one true food friend, my one constant comfort was always sugar. Sweets were the friend that would never let me down. Part of the problem was that sweet, sugary treats were used as a reward in our family, so my father was always bringing home sweets of one sort or another. Case in point: the day my period started, my dad came home with a cake to celebrate. Thank God it didn't say "HAPPY PE-RIOD!" on it, but it did have red roses made of frosting, and I ate most of that cake while thinking it marked the start of me becoming a woman. I was twelve years old, but even then I knew I'd need a lot more than cake to comfort me on the journey to womanhood.

Looking back, I wouldn't say I had a bad childhood. My family was middle class, we went on fun vacations, and we had a nice house and a pool. The only thing that makes the memories hard to look back on is the way I always felt about myself: something was very, very wrong with me. Something everyone could see. Something I couldn't hide, something the doctors, the nutritionists, and my parents couldn't fix…and it was getting worse every single day.

I think at some point I just accepted my new reality: I was always going to be fat—I was Fat Jasinda. So I made a decision: if I was always going to have this problem, then I'd better have smarts, talent, and humor to make up for it. So one day I started talking to God about how we could make this happen. I decided I was going to grow up to be a rock star, a chubby Tiffany or Debbie Gibson. It would be my destiny. So, in the name of taking charge of my life, that day I marched into my room with a box of Pop Tarts and started practicing.

Chapter 2

BEING A FAT ADULT ALSO SUCKS

"What can I say? I've never met a cupcake I didn't want to get to know better."—Anna, *Big Girls Do It Better* by Jasinda Wilder

I WAS ACTUALLY PRETTY POPULAR IN HIGH SCHOOL—I KNOW, I know, it was pretty shocking to me, too. I kept myself busy in band, choir and drama. I was a nerdy, academic, popular fat kid. I was in all the school plays and musicals—usually as the mom or the funny wife of a secondary character, but at least I got a part. I also helped with the production and choreography for the show choir, and I kept dancing through everything. During this time I was accepted to, and attended, a very prestigious summer arts program where I studied vocal arts.

At the time, I weighed over three hundred pounds, probably closer to three-thirty, but I managed to keep active and I stayed busy all the time. My grades were pretty good, and I was even in some honors classes.

Things were…survivable.

I had my first boyfriend around that time—I won't go into much detail to protect the innocent, but I will say things could have been worse. He wasn't the type of boy your parents would pick out for you. He was rough around the edges, to say the least. Although that little relationship didn't last very long, it did give my self-esteem a tiny boost, and I was able to lose about forty pounds before my high school graduation.

I was kicking life's ass!

Then, near the end of my senior year of high school, I went to a party. I was a goody-goody, keep in mind, so I never really got into any trouble. That night, though, I decided to experiment with alcohol for the first time, and I ended up blacking out. I have no solid proof, but I believe I was sexually assaulted that night.

And, of course, I subconsciously blamed what had happened on my recent weight loss: I had let my guard down, I had been stupid—but I wouldn't be making *that* mistake again. I vowed I would only succumb to food in the future.

Cue the dramatic music.

I had applied to the music departments of several colleges even though I wasn't really sure where to go with my music. Ultimately, I attended the university that offered me a full ride. My parents told me that that sort of scholarship wasn't something you should turn down, so I agreed and packed my bags.

At the time, my music career was going very well; I was doing gigs and singing at weddings, funerals, and paid community events almost every weekend. I even talked with a record producer about doing a demo for a label but, in the end, I decided I was more of a teacher than a performer. Also, I wanted to have a fallback plan in place, since everybody knows you don't make money with an arts degree. So Michigan State's music education program seemed like a good choice.

Let me tell you, Michigan State University was a pretty crazy place when I was there. Remember the riots? I was there when they were burning couches, and students were getting run over by fire trucks—those things happened literally right outside my dorm room window. I spent way too many nights hiding in my closet, either from the rioting or from the graphic sounds of my roommate and her boyfriend having sex.

Two very important events occurred that first year of university: I started dating a boy from my hometown who had graduated high school the year before me, so we had several mutual friends in common. And then, during my first year at MSU, right around Christmas, my parents called and told me they were separating.

My parents always seemed to have a wonderful relationship, so I didn't understand why they were separating, or how they could live apart. My dad was now living with my grandparents and my mom was "going away" for the holidays. My whole world spun upside down. My parents had always seemed happy. I never even saw them fight much. I couldn't comprehend what was happening. This news was a huge blow to me, leaving me in total shock.

So what did I do? I turned to my old friend Food for comfort. She had always been there for me before, and I knew she wouldn't let me down now.

In less than two months I had: a) quit school and transferred to a college closer to home, b) gained back all the weight I'd lost, and c) told the new boyfriend I would marry him.

Which decision do you think was the worst for me? If you guessed d) all of the above, you would be correct.

I'll spare you all the gory, painful details, but the relationship went downhill fast. I should have known it was a bad idea to get married when, on the day of the nuptials, the wedding arrangement that arrived at the church was, in fact, a funeral arrangement. True story!

Our relationship became physically violent very soon after the wedding. And shortly after that I became very, very depressed: my husband was never home, I was lonely, and my parents were still working on repairing their marriage. I was lonely and bored—I was still going to school and working part time, but I just wasn't fulfilled by any of those things.

So I started eating.

And I ate a *lot*.

I ate all the time.

I ate horrible, awful foods crammed full of sugar.

I quickly ballooned up to over 400 pounds, and was suddenly hit with a barrage of medical problems. Erratic periods, a resurgence of asthma, problems with my feet, skin rashes, problems sleeping, snoring…you name it, I had it. It was a dark and scary time for me. I quit my classes and my job. I stayed at home and sat in my house and ate. Food was my only friend.

I endured not one, not two, but *three* miscarriages in a very short space of time. The doctor told me the weight of my body was just too much for the pregnancies to be viable. It was quite possible I had PCOS, Polycystic Ovary Syndrome. I began taking anti-depressants just to make the anxiety manageable.

I'd given up.

Because all I did was watch TV, I dreamed of Jerry Springer having to cut me out of my house because I was getting so big, which wasn't too far from reality. While watching one of my mid-day shows, I saw a commercial for bariatric surgery. It sounded interesting. Maybe this was how I could solve all my problems at once. I was already suffering with an enormous amount of physical pain, so surely cutting myself open from top to bottom and radically changing the processes of my internal organs couldn't be that much more painful, could it?

I figured if I had to choose between a quick death from surgery, and a slow death from eating too much, then it might be better to just try the surgery, right?

I picked up the phone and made the call.

At that point, I didn't think I had much to lose.

Chapter 3

WEIGHT LOSS SURGERY AND OTHER HUGE MISTAKES

A<small>T THIS POINT</small> I <small>WAS</small> 20 <small>YEARS OLD WITH NO COLLEGE DEGREE,</small> severe depression, an abusive husband, and I was morbidly obese. I felt as if the only way I could fix everything was to undergo gastric bypass surgery.

Before you start making any assumptions, let me tell you I investigated this surgery very thoroughly before I had it done. I researched online, joined a forum, talked to my doctors, went to a support group, and spoke with several different surgeons.

I was told my internal organs were beginning to shut down, one by one, because of my weight. I was also told I might never be able to have children, and that I was starting to show signs of diabetes—a condition I had watched my grandmother suffer from my whole life.

This surgery seemed like a magic solution to all my problems. If only I could get this weight off, everything would be better! I would want to live! I would have the will power to turn things around, this time for good! Food would no longer rule me!

It sounded like the perfect plan.

So, with a physiological evaluation under my belt, on the day before my 21st birthday I had a full RNY gastric bypass surgery. I woke up in pain, and was given drugs. I don't remember much about the first few days after my surgery, but I do remember being given chicken broth, Jell-O and popsicles, but I didn't want any of them.

I now had a giant scar that went from just under my breastbone all the way down to my pubic bone. I couldn't look at myself in the mirror, because it all looked just too awful. My scars were more than just reminders of the surgery; they stood as stark proof of my desperation, evidence of so much emotional pain.

I lost two hundred pounds in what seemed like overnight, although it obviously took longer than that. I didn't really want to eat at all that first year, mostly because it was simply too painful; food had now become the enemy and my body was winning the war. I got down to a size fourteen, but I still felt sick inside. I still didn't like the way I looked. I still wasn't comfortable in my skin.

Shouldn't I be happier now?

I was still struggling emotionally, yet, because I was thinner, my confidence increased a bit. What a strange conflict, right?

So, with my newfound confidence I began singing again, and I began working as a karaoke DJ. As well, I taught vocal lessons on the weekend. Physically, I was starting to make tiny steps back into the world, but I was still completely lost mentally and emotionally. My husband grew more and more distant. He worked all the time and, when he was home, he was unhappy. The one small connection we'd shared was food, but I no longer wanted to eat. He became angry and suspicious of the people I was working with. He became increasingly violent towards me, and our relationship only ended when he went to jail. I can't really place all the blame on him, even though I probably should. I was a mess, and we both were very, very young.

My body had changed—*I* had changed.

I decided to have some plastic surgery done to remove my excess skin. I thought that would help improve my self-image and make my clothes fit better; it seemed like a win/win to me. Yes, the physical pain from the surgery would be tough, but I had been through that before and I figured I could do it again. I had blocked out most of the memories of that experience anyway.

After this surgery, however, I ended up getting a horrible infection, which nearly killed me. I spent weeks in the hospital having the wound reopened over and over in an attempt to rid my body of the infection. When the hospital called my husband to ask him if he would come and be with me, he refused. He was done with my mess. Heck, *I* was done with my mess. It certainly doesn't excuse his physical violence toward me—nothing ever will—but in my mind it helps me understand, just a little.

Marriage is difficult enough to begin with, but when you don't love yourself it becomes almost impossible. I didn't see it then, but somewhere in all the mess and complications of life, I had stopped loving myself. I had given up. I was probably as close to death as you could be without actually dying.

I moved back in with my parents—who, thankfully, had reconciled by this point—got divorced, kept working, and started dating. I figured if I had this new body, I might as well use it, right? I really wasn't into having sex, but making out sounded pretty fun. I still had trouble eating and I was continuing to lose weight. I supported myself by working almost exclusively in bars, either singing or DJing.

And that's when Chase walked into the bar one night and began singing.

(As a quick aside, if you haven't read the *Big Girls Do It* series, you should probably put this book down real quick and pick that one up, just so you can get all the juicy details of my life at that time. Yes, Chase and Jeff are based on real-life love interests. I was just trying to figure out whom I was and what I wanted to do and, at the same time, pay my bills. In the books, I rewrote history a little, and chose Jeff for Anna pretty much right off the bat, whereas in real life Anna was with Chase a bit longer.)

Okay, back to the narrative.

When I was pregnant with my oldest son, we found out when he was born that he'd suffered with IUGR (intrauterine growth restriction), and my daughter, who followed soon after, had the same problem. After the birth of my daughter I got so sick that I couldn't get out of bed, and I bled intensely for a long, long time, hemorrhaging from basically everywhere. I saw specialist after specialist, but no one could tell me what was wrong.

The diagnosis I received from the first two doctors was that I had leukemia, and a third doctor suggested colon cancer. I was horrified! Here I was, a mother with two little babies. I couldn't die! I went to the best hematologist-oncologist I could find, and when I met with him after having my blood tested, he told me that my hemoglobin was at a two—a normal hemoglobin result is between twelve and fifteen. Something was terribly wrong with me, but he didn't think it was leukemia, which gave me a little comfort at least, but not much. He took samples of my blood and sent it to the Mayo Clinic for analysis. They sent it back saying it wasn't real blood, so we took more samples and sent them in. Again, they said my samples couldn't possibly be blood: these samples had zero nutrients. Zip. Zero. None of the nutrients contained in normal blood were present in mine. I was walking death.

I remember calling my good friend after the appointment and telling her I was probably going to die. Not only was she a wonderful mentor, friend, and counselor to me, but she was also a prayer partner. We prayed together that night and in my head I started planning my own funeral. I know this sounds grim, but that was how things looked at the time.

Together we prayed for a miracle.

This was a very difficult time for me, but I promise things are going to turn around with this story soon. Please stick with me—there's a light at the end of the tunnel.

Chapter 4

PREGNANCY AND OTHER WEIRD SHIT THAT REALLY EFFED UP MY BODY

I BEGAN TO REALIZE WHAT I'D DONE TO MYSELF, AND I BECAME angry. And this is where all that shit became horribly real.

By the time I finally received a correct diagnosis, I was virtually unable to leave my bed. I was weak to the point that I couldn't take care of my kids. I was pale, I was losing my hair, and I was continually bleeding. It was a nightmare. The diagnosis was a non-nutrient blood disorder caused by the gastric bypass.

I had tried to save myself…by nearly killing myself. Again.

The surgeon who performed the bypass admitted he might have removed too much intestinal and stomach tissue, figuring that because of my height more was better. At that point, however, it was too risky to fix the problems with my stomach and intestines, so my doctors decided to insert a medical port into my chest so they could infuse my blood with nutrients.

The surgery to insert the port didn't happen without its own complications, though, because this is *me* we're talking about here. The operating room was overbooked the day of the procedure so, to save time, they tried to give me a twilight sleep—a lighter anesthetic that my body didn't accept. I woke up during the procedure and pan-icked, but I was physically immobile and unable to alert the surgeons that I was awake and feeling everything they were doing. Obviously I survived, but it's an experience I wouldn't wish on my worst enemy.

The port itself is still in place, eight years later, and it is still working. One of my goals for myself with this program is to become healthy enough so that I no longer need the port, and I can have it removed.

When I first had the port, I needed medication infused almost daily. Fortunately, I was able to get a home healthcare nurse who came and helped me with these daily infusions. It was amazingly helpful having her come to my house every day because, honestly, I was still feeling too weak to even leave my bed. She was a sweet, won-derful lady and she took great care of me. She really did help me heal both my body and my soul during an excruciatingly hard time in my life. I cried many tears as she listened and gave me my medicine.

My friends and my church group continued to pray for me, and soon I was feeling better and was able to get back to work teaching, leading worship, and being a wife and mother. My body was some-times able to store enough nutrients that I could go days or even weeks without needing an infusion, but it was a constant balancing act between managing the frequent blood-work results and the med-ication.

I just want to take a moment here to say that my heart, and my thanks, goes out to all the nurses out there who take care of the hurt-ing, the hopeless, and those in pain. Yours is not an easy job and it can be thankless at times, but I know I wouldn't be here without you. You inspire me with your kind, compassionate hearts.

In 2010 I got pregnant again and my doctors, now knowing what happens with my body during pregnancy, were very proactive about getting nutrients into my body. I had a high-risk specialist, constant ultra-sounds, and regular infusions to make sure both the baby and I were healthy. My pregnancy was very happy and I was healthy. I gained lots of weight, but my baby did too, and that was my primary concern. He came at the end of November, looking like a stuffed Thanksgiving turkey. I was so proud of what my body had accomplished!

And then, just a few months after having him, I got pregnant *again*, which came as a huge shock to me. Yes, I *do* know how babies are made—and I happen to enjoy that part, thank you very much! —but we were on birth control and I just wasn't expecting to have any more kids.

My body never really had enough time to recover between pregnancies, so that pregnancy was a rough one. Once again the doctors took great care of me and the baby. We had frequent ultra-sounds and I was still taking my medication regularly, but the simple fact was that I just wasn't ready to be pregnant again. My body was *so* tired. I know all you mamas out there who have had babies back-to-back will understand what I'm saying. Having a baby is like a marathon: if you don't get that recovery time after the birth, you just aren't going to recover properly.

It's weird, because even though those two pregnancies were so close together, the boys are so very different from each other. After my fourth child I felt so refreshed, energized, even, but after my fifth I felt as if I wasn't ever going to recover.

And then, two weeks after he was born, baby number five contracted RSV—respiratory syncytial virus. He was born a few weeks early, so the virus hit him hard. I knew something was wrong when

I saw him turn blue. We rushed to the hospital where they took one look at him and put him on a respirator. He was so small, and so sick. I can still see his tiny little hands and feet turning blue, and my husband holding him and praying to God, begging Him not to take our sweet baby that He let him stay with us.

Neither of us slept much while our son was in the hospital. I think I managed *maybe* five or six hours of sleep that whole first week. It got to the point that my father and husband had to haul me literally kicking and screaming from the hospital and put me into a car with my friend who took me home so I could rest. I was worried my son would die if I took even a few minutes to sleep. My friend came to pray over me while I slept, the same amazing friend who'd prayed with me after my plastic surgery, a time when I was sure I was going to die.

If you saw our CBS interview you know that at that time my husband was in an honors teaching program, which we had struggled for years to put him through. My teaching income barely kept us at poverty level, even after adding in his student loans, so needless to say things were tight. Jack had to take days, and then weeks, off from the program, some of which he had already missed because of the birth. While our son was in the hospital, Jack got a call from the university telling him that he had forty-eight hours to return to the program, or he'd be cut from it. We knew that based on how the classes were set up that if he left he might never get back into that program again. They were extremely selective, and even if he were re-accepted, we'd have to wait another whole year to reapply. That same night our son took yet another turn for the worse. We decided then that Jack just couldn't return to the program—he couldn't even bear to leave the hospital.

We weren't sure how we would move forward with this news but we did know that we needed to focus on getting our son healthy and back at home. It was—and remains to this day—the most difficult time of our lives.

I still can't think about that time without choking up—my computer screen is blurring from tears as I write these words. Our son did recover and was able to come home with us after two weeks in the hospital. He's now healthy and happy, and he is our sweet but crazy little wild man, and we simply cannot fathom our lives without his cute, impish grin and devious ways.

So by now I'm sure you're probably thinking, "Gosh, these first few chapters have all been pretty depressing."

I promise you there's a silver lining in all of this.

Jack, who was no longer in the teaching program, had to come up with a way to help support our family, because without the student loans to supplement my income, things weren't just tight for us anymore, but completely unsustainable. We *had* to do something.

We happened to stumble upon an article about self-publishing and, as they say, the rest is history. We began writing and ended up with several *New York Times*, *USA TODAY*, and *Wall Street Journal* bestselling novels. I could easily spend a few chapters on this subject, but I think I'll save it for a book on my marriage with my husband somewhere down the road.

The important thing is that we survived, we thrived, and we got my health issues mostly under control. We got busy writing, attending signings, and raising our family.

Today, we wake up every single day feeling so blessed, not so much because we have enough money to feed everyone—which is both important and comforting—but more because we get to do what we love: tell stories, entertain, and inspire.

I believe all that struggle and pain has been for a reason. It might have even have led me to be able to write this book, using my own experiences to inspire and help others going through similar situations. Sometimes, when I look back on those times and compare them to where I'm at now, it really does seem as if it was a different person who experienced all that pain.

Many of you reading this book have been following us since reading our first book, so you know our story. Heck, you could probably write it better than me! But these chapters are important because you need to know where I'm coming from, especially when we get into the next part of my story. You'll come to understand that I'm a woman just like you and, like many of you; I've been through some shit. I've put my body through so much stress and so much hell. I've tried everything to heal myself—and I mean *everything*—from nasty pills that made me poop raw fat to countless painful workout videos. I'm someone who has given up so many times, and who has been given countless second, third, and fourth chances. I've failed more than I've succeeded. But I'm a survivor.

Health wise, things began to change for me during my most recent pregnancy. I don't know how or why, but I started to *lose* weight, which was very, very strange. We also learned that two people in our immediate families had been diagnosed with diabetes. That was a HUGE revelation for me. I started getting really angry, and when I get angry, I do something about it.

I began to research like a madwoman. I've always read a lot of non-fiction, and health and wellness books in particular, but because of the revelations I was experiencing and the changes I was feeling in my body, my research really cranked up to a possibly obsessive level. I had to know why my body was acting so differently. Why did I feel so different during this pregnancy, and how could I continue to feel this way after the baby was born? I wanted to be healthy for my husband, my kids, and myself.

I didn't want to continue to feel as if every day was a struggle. I didn't want to feel like I was dying inside.

I wanted to be truly healthy. I wanted to live, and live well!

PART 2:

My Favorite Part of the Story

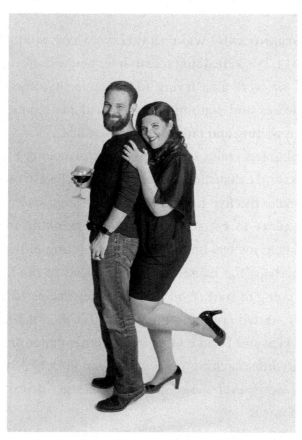

Chapter 5:

OOPS, WE DID IT AGAIN!

MY HUSBAND AND I WERE TRAVELING A LOT DURING THE FALL of 2014. We were doing research for a new book on Mackinac Island, and we were also trying to schedule in some down time between releases and signings, and we had just come back from speaking at a writing and publishing conference.

I started to feel really, really sick on the plane, but I just chalked it up to stress and exhaustion. When we landed I wasn't sure I would be able to make the five-hour car journey home, so we stopped at a shopping plaza to get something to eat, thinking maybe some food would help me feel better. As we were sitting in the restaurant I thought perhaps the nausea could be related to the fact that my period was going to start. *Wait, when was my last period?* I couldn't remember. I started counting the weeks and then it hit me: a few weeks back Jack and I had had an *oops* moment after one too many Stella Artois while watching *The Fault In Our Stars*. Yep, it had been a kids-should-never-ever-die-of-cancer-so-let's-get-drunk-and-have-crazy-sex moment.

I started hyper ventilating—I was completely freaking out. There was no way in heck we could be having a baby! I literally ran into Target, grabbed a pregnancy test, darted into the bathroom, and peed on the stick right then and there. After a few minutes of waiting and freaking out I got the results…and then I sent my husband a text message screenshot of the positive test.

HOLY SHIT! We were having a baby.

Now, please understand, I really do believe every child is a blessing, but I really only ever set out to have two…and now I was going to have *SIX*? Life can be pretty freaking crazy.

I spent the rest of the ride home sucking on peppermints, crying, and breathing into a paper bag. In the back of my mind I was sure this was God's way of slowing us down. I'd been feeling like all the business travel we were doing was worsening my health, and my lab results were proving me right. Maybe this news was an easy way for us to re-group and take some much-needed time to be with our family, and just relax for a change. Right? Um… if you know us, you're probably laughing (I'm sure my agent is) but, honestly, it was my happy thought to hold on to: a baby would bring downtime and rest. Ha!

Once we got home I called my OB/GYN because I knew she would want to see me right away, given my crazy health history. When I went to the appointment a few weeks later they wanted to weigh me. Now, what you have to understand is I had basically given up on weighing myself, to the point that I didn't even *own* a scale. I just didn't want to know, because I always ended up feeling sad and angry. There was no controlling my weight, just the depressing reality that the numbers would just keep going up no matter what I did. I wasn't even really trying to diet anymore. My weight would go up and down with my menstrual cycle, and arbitrarily, as well. I had been told that my blood nutrient disorder and the other nutritional issues that developed as a result of the bypass would make it nearly impossible for me to lose any substantial amount weight. My body chemistry was behaving as if I was starving, so it would hold onto the bad stuff and release the good before I could absorb any nutrients from the food. I was trying to eat mostly healthy foods, but I did have sweets occasionally and I wasn't counting calories, or being very physically active. When we weren't at home, I was sitting most of the day while travelling, or sitting trying to finish whatever book we were working on. At home I sometimes used my walking tread-mill desk, but it wasn't enough. I was mostly sedentary, apart from the occasional ride on my trusty horse Cowboy.

The nurse insisted she get a weight reading from me, and I grimaced at the *319* pounds that appeared on the readout when I stepped onto the scale. There was no way I could have gained that much! When the hell did that happen? Who had been stuffing all that fat into my ass? My OB said she wanted to keep a watch on my weight, and scheduled me for a few tests. I left feeling both excited and worried. I really needed my body to work well for this pregnancy, because I knew this was going to be my last baby, and I wanted to be as healthy as I could for him or her. I prayed that God would help me be strong through this pregnancy, both mentally and physically. I needed to find my health. I was on a mission.

That night, I dreamed of a laughing baby girl.

Most of my life hasn't gone as planned; in fact, it usually goes total-ly contrary to anything I plan. This pregnancy was unplanned, and the results of the pregnancy equally so. Initially, our older children weren't that excited about having a new sibling—remember, they had to deal with two mischievous toddler brothers, and now we were having *another* baby. The first thing they said when we told them was that we would have to get a bigger car. This really upset them because we had just purchased a lovely 7-seat SUV that they all really liked. Nonetheless, the idea of another sibling seemed to grow on them, and by mid-pregnancy they were showing some signs of excitement.

My daughter requested the baby be a girl because we already had WAY too much testosterone in our house. There's a more equal gender ratio in the barn, so she likes to stay out there as much as she can. Don't get me wrong, she can hang with the boys, but she would much rather spend time with her pony, Shorty. She convinced the boys to start praying for a girl too, because they were already sharing a room and adding one more boy would mean fewer toys and less space for them. I just wanted a healthy, happy mama and baby. Since I'd had so many complications with my previous pregnancies, health was my number one goal for both of us.

Around the second trimester I started feeling pretty good. I wasn't overly exhausted and I was finally able to keep most of my food down. We were dealing with some work stress, which wasn't unusual, but overall I felt the pregnancy was going pretty well. At my 4th or 5th month appointment my OB remarked that I was losing some weight, and we both figured it was due to the fact that I had had so much nausea early on in the pregnancy. She told me not to worry too much about it, the baby was measuring normal, so I was just to continue eating as healthily as I could.

Once I reached the halfway point in the pregnancy, my entire outlook on food changed. It was sudden and it was drastic. Anything containing sugar immediately turned my stomach. It was a very strange reaction to what had been my comfort food, my long-time best friend. I remember our sweet nanny making the kids a special after-school treat and she asked me to try it. I took one bite and spit it out; I just couldn't tolerate the sweetness even though everyone else raved about it. Weird things were happening to me.

The second odd thing that happened was my reaction to my normal morning breakfast. For about three years my breakfast has consisted of toast and yogurt—a peach Chobani yogurt to be exact. As the pregnancy went on I started to get light headed after eating. This really became a problem when I would try to shower after breakfast and would have to get out of the shower and sit down, trying to not pass out.

It took me weeks to figure out that what I was eating was somehow connected to how I was feeling.

I'm sure moms out there are wondering about gestational diabetes. I had done a fasting blood work panel and all of my levels had come back totally normal, so this dizziness was really bizarre. Again, as I have previously stated, *nothing* about my body has ever made sense and nothing ever goes as planned. At my next checkup, the scale once again revealed that I was continuing to lose weight. We had another ultrasound planned for the baby, and as long as that looked okay my OB said things would be fine. Everything looked good on the ultrasound with Baby Wilder, so we just chalked the dizziness up to my weird nutrient levels and the pregnancy.

By springtime, my family and friends were starting to notice that I was losing weight. The difference in my face was pretty drastic—the previous roundness was now more sculpted, and my eyes looked bigger. My clothes were starting to get baggy, and the only way to tell I was pregnant was to look directly at my belly with my shirt pulled up. This was unlike every other pregnancy. What was going on with my body? It was a mystery.

Right around that same time, two people in our immediate families were diagnosed with diabetes. My husband had already been dealing with some blood sugar issues at his young age of 33. Diabetes ran on both my side of the family and his which meant our kids had an even greater chance of developing it, as well.

I began a quest for answers and started doing some research. Now, I know it's common knowledge that I'm a pretty fast typist, but I'm not sure how much I've spoken about how fast I read. Well, I started devouring one or two non-fiction books per day on diabetes, nutrition, exercise, and overall health. I was also Googling like mad, trying to figure out if the changes to my body were mental, emotional, chemical, or just physical. Maybe, after 35 years, my body was just done with the way I had been eating, and maybe it had decided to take things into its own hands?

My research kept bringing me back to one primary culprit: my good old friend sugar. I started thinking back on my childhood and those damn angel food cakes. Apart from those cakes, what *had* I eaten back then? Weight Watcher® meals, Healthy Choice pre-packaged meals, diet bars, diet soda… I started to take a closer look at those things.

Man, I had been eating *junk*!

It was almost too depressing to even think about. But my mindset was changing. Now I was really focused on the idea of food being fuel. It was no longer working as simply a comfort or a friend to me. I wanted/needed the right fuels to keep my sweet baby and myself going strong. So what changed? What was so different now? I asked myself these questions and made a list:

- I didn't want to die prematurely. For me, this had always been a frightening and constant reality simply because of my weight alone. Yes, weighing 430 pounds was actually slowing killing me. And then, once I had the bypass and lost some weight, the blood disorder I developed became a constant threat to my life. Despite my infusions and medications, and the fact that I was usually able to keep a good handle on things, it was still very scary for my family and me.

- I was done dieting—I was *beyond* done dieting.
- I was done being unsuccessful. I hated being a bad example for my kids, and I hated being so negative about my body and my health. Yes, I tried to keep a positive self-image and body-image both at home and professionally but, let's face it, it's hard not feeling well *all the time*. I was often tired, and I wanted to be active and to just, basically…*feel good*.
- I was thinking about my body differently.
- Things just didn't taste the same. I know you've heard the old saying "nothing tastes as good as skinny feels." Well, for me it had become "nothing tastes as good as healthy feels." I had reached a point where my health had become my main priority.

My own health and the health of my family became my primary focus. I was determined to turn things around and I knew it would all start with food. I have more on the specifics later in the book, but there were two things that I think made the biggest impact on my health and body during my pregnancy: cutting out sugar, and starting my day with protein—specifically farm fresh eggs.

Sounds fairly easy right?

Well, during my pregnancy it sort of was. I think most people would think that cutting out sugar would be the hardest part, but because I was feeling such adverse affects from sugar during my pregnancy, it was pretty easy for me to eliminate it. All in all I lost about

30 pounds during my pregnancy. It was both strange and beautiful, and I embraced the ease of my weight loss…and then the baby came and all hell broke loose.

Chapter 6

AND THEN CAME JOYFUL NUMBER SIX

I'VE REALLY GOT TO COMMEND OUR NEW SWEET BABY GIRL FOR really rolling with the punches, because she was born into a crazy circus of a family. Most babies probably wouldn't choose to join a household with five other kids, two crazy *New York Times* bestselling workaholic parents, and 100 farm animals. Well… maybe they might. We do have some pretty cool mini-donkeys.

All joking aside, sweet Ree came into the world on June 30, 2015, right when she wanted to, the only one of my children to ever go past their due date. She came out smiling and hasn't stopped since. She loves to eat and sleep, and smile and smile and smile. Sometimes I worry that her poor little face is going to crack because she is always smiling so big. Had all of my babies been like her, we would probably have a dozen.

We had about one hour of peace with her before all hell broke loose. First, someone hit our car in the parking lot of the hospital while I was giving birth, a hit and run. Then we got an email from our editor informing us that our edits needed to be turned in to Berkley, our new traditional publishing partner, within a week's time, which was a lot sooner than we'd thought. And *then* we found out we were being audited by the IRS! Yay!

No kidding—this was all within days of bringing our new baby home from the hospital.

Can you guess what happened? The stress of it all caused me to spiral downwards, and *fast*. I ended up depressed and comforting myself with food. Yep, my old friend was back. Within a few weeks I had put on ten pounds. Here I was with this beautiful, perfect, smiling baby and I was feeling like a bloated, stressed out bag of mommy poop.

Who's got the wine?

I spent a good week or so wallowing in my own self-pity and more than a few bottles of wine. We got the car fixed, the edits done, a CPA dealing with the IRS, and I was looking forward to seeing some of my author friends who were coming into town for a signing. As good as it would be to see them, I was still feeling really crappy, and if you know my beautiful and amazing friends Tara Sivec and R.K. Lilley, you know they are as sweet as they are gorgeous. Well, hanging around those two beauties only ended up making me feel even angrier with myself. I was *done* with the way things were going.

Let me just say, as an aside, that post partum depression is no joke. Ladies, if you are feeling down for any reason after giving birth to your precious little baby PLEASE talk to someone, although it probably shouldn't be your mother or your husband, but rather a friend or a medical professional who can be more objective, someone who can help you get perspective, or help, and/or medication. There is such a stigma regarding mental health in general and depression in particular in our country. Postpartum depression a very real thing, and left untreated it can ruin mothers, and fracture families. Please get help when you need it, because that new little life needs you happy and healthy.

Ok, now that I've gotten that out of the way, back to my story.

The Monday after my friends left, I took a picture of myself in the mirror, wearing only my bra and underwear. It was a "come to Jesus" moment for me, let me tell you. I realized I had only two choices: either I could continue on as I had been for the past 30 years, or I could fight back. For the second time in my life I knew I didn't have much to lose; I was going to fight.

My precious baby girl had been the key to weight loss during my pregnancy, and I was going to use her as my motivation again—I wanted to live a long and healthy life with her. I didn't want to feel sick anymore. There *had* to be a way to get this shit under control.

So I pulled up my good friend Google and got to work trying to figure out a plan I could manage long-term which would also be successful for my whole family. I knew that if I was going to be healthier we would all need to do this together, which meant that somehow I had to get everyone on board with it. All five of the older kids *and* my husband would need to see why these changes had to happen, and understand why I needed them to support my plan.

I had been blind for so long to many of the health issues in our family, and my research was telling me they were all being aggravated—if not outright *caused*—by the food we were eating. My family has ADHD, autism spectrum disorder, asthma, food allergy and sensitivity, and constipation, just to name a few. I came up with an action plan.

I sat down with my family and I laid it all out for them.

We were going to eat as healthily as possible, and we were going to be more physically active. I wanted to teach them how to decide day by day, meal by meal, what the best foods were to put in their bodies, and I would teach them by example. I was doing it for them, but I was also doing it for myself and maybe even for future generations.

See, when I was a child I was fed a steaming load of bullshit about what I should be eating, which has negatively affected me my whole life. I believe now that what I had been told to eat were actually the things that made me so unhealthy. These same foods had actually *caused* the majority my heath problems, directly and indirectly. I'm not trying to shift blame—I know my parents did the best they could to help me, I just think the so-called "experts" they had trusted were flat-out wrong. I think the diet and the food industry were wrong, and I believe that my desperation was fueled by those bad eating decisions. It had been a perfect storm and now I was determined to do everything I could to steer my kids away from that.

I was jumping on the bandwagon of parents who made family health a priority. Yeah, I admit it; I sometimes rolled my eyes at those moms who went around requesting "healthy snacks" for their kids at school. Those crazy, homemade-baby-food-making, grain-grinding mamas who got up early in the morning to prep meals. Yeah, *those* crazy mamas. I was turning into one of them.

I just *knew* my family would love this idea.

Chapter 7

MAKING THE PLAN

"I am a better person when I have less on my plate."
— Elizabeth Gilbert, author of *Eat, Pray, Love*

IF YOU WERE TO GO A BOOKSTORE OR DO A SEARCH ON AMAZON right now, you'd find roughly three trillion books on diet, health, and fitness by a variety of so-called and self-proclaimed "experts". As I pointed out in the foreword at the beginning of this book, I am not in any way, shape, or form an expert—I just want to share with you the things that have worked fairly easily and quickly for my family and me. Now, "easily and quickly" is a relative term, and I certainly don't want to market this book as some sort of magical get-skinny-quick scheme. If anything, nothing could be further from the truth.

What I'm going to lay out for you is what worked for us. It might work for you, but it might not, or not in the same way it did our family. From my research, though, my guess is that our plan will help more people than I could even begin to estimate at this moment.

My plan is fairly straightforward, even allowing for the fact that our family has children from under one year of age to twelve years old, with very picky toddlers in the mix. I had to make sure the plan allowed every member of my family not just to survive and be healthy, but to thrive, enjoy life, and enjoy food.

As I mentioned, the first thing I did was call a big family meeting. I should point out before we go any further, however, that my biggest worry when calling this meeting was actually my husband. If you know Jack at all you know he is very vocal about his hatred of all vegetables. So much so, in fact, that if you ever get him drinking he'll tell you about the time he held lima beans in his mouth for several hours rather than swallow them. It was only after his mother discovered them still half-chewed inside his mouth *three hours* after he left the table that she sent him to go and spit them all out. Obviously, Jack *hates* lima beans, but he also shudders with disgust when I bring up nasty words like broccoli or cauliflower. The struggle is real—just ask his mother.

Jack's aversion to vegetables led to the crux of the problem: I knew for this plan to work, we needed to incorporate a lot more leafy greens and veggies into our diet. I can almost hear mothers everywhere laughing as they are reading this: yeah, right—mothers have been trying to get their families to eat vegetables since the beginning of time. Well, I was going to give it my best shot…I had to either get them past Jack or hide them so he couldn't figure out what he was eating.

But first I got everyone into the family huddle and talked to them about my health, and how I had decided now was the time to choose health, and that I was going to make as many healthy choices in my life as I could. My sweet little three year-old just kept nodding his little head, and my nine year-old daughter was rolling her eyes and thinking, "Oh boy, here we go. Mom's lost her mind."

I explained the basics of diabetes to them, and told them the disease ran on both my side of the family *and* Daddy's, and that two of our family members were already struggling to manage it. I told them I felt it was my responsibility as their mother to help them be as healthy as they could be. I told them I loved them, and that I wanted them to live long and healthy lives.

I could tell about half the group had totally tuned out and were thinking about which TV show they were going to watch after dinner, but at least two of the children were at least somewhat interested in what I was saying. Jack was playing his usual supportive husband role, but I hadn't got to the part about vegetables.

The kids wanted to know what this would mean, and how would it change the way we actually ate. Would there be gross stuff? Would we have to stop going out to dinner? Could they still have cookies?

I answered their questions as best as I could, but I didn't want to drop too many bombs on them right away—I knew from experience it was best to ease them into things. No need to scare them, right?

So, when they woke up the next day, instead of their usual breakfast of toast, cereal, or granola bars, I told them they could have either some Greek yogurt or some eggs. I hadn't picked those items at random, however; there was a reason behind these choices. I'd been researching a lot and really felt that if we were going to kick our sugar habit, then we needed to start the day off loaded with protein. My plan was to start by changing our breakfast choices, and then I would change dinner, and then hopefully lunch would come on its own.

The first two days were a bit rough. The younger ones weren't sure about the options I'd given them; they really wanted their usual cereal—which weren't even the really bad sugary ones like Lucky Charms or Cap'n Crunch—rice puffs and Cheerios, mostly. They weren't necessarily horrible, but they weren't the best choices either.

I know, I know. Cheerios? How can Cheerios be bad for you? Keep reading and you'll see what I'm talking about.

By the end of week one I was already starting to see changes in everyone. Real, noticeable changes! I had so much more energy than before, my clothes were feeling looser, and I wasn't bloated, two of my kids noticed a decrease in their constipation and insomnia... and this was *week one*. Things were changing just from switching up our breakfast options! I knew I was on to something. If just this small change could have such a huge impact, what effects would other changes have?

Next, I was going to get rid of all the juice and pop in the house. I just *knew* my family would be on board enthusiastically with that too, right? Seriously, I knew it wouldn't be easy but I had to try, because soda, diet or regular, is a killer, no exaggeration. My older kids only had soda on rare occasions, maybe two or three cans a week at most, but after all of my research I knew any at all was terrible for them. What about juice? Well, the amount of sugar in things like apple juice is much less than in soda, but even too much fructose can be bad.

I had to find a way to lure them into creating healthy habits.

I decided to find fun replacements for the bubbly, sugary drinks they wanted. My first pick was LaCroix brand naturally flavored water. The great thing about LaCroix is they aren't much more expensive than soda, they have a really wide variety of flavors, and the cans come in really bright, bold colors—which may seem silly, but it's a well known fact in the marketing industry that colorful packaging is extremely important. I bought a couple of different flavors, and I was honestly surprised at how easy it was to get them to drink those.

We also bought a few different flavors of Stevia-sweetened "soda"—which is really just sparkling water with a bit of added sweetness to it, so it tastes closer to real soda. Those went over even better; my kids really enjoy the orange, grape, cream soda, and root beer flavors. These beverages are also free of the added colors and dyes regular sodas contain.

Finally, we bought True Lemon and True Lime—don't worry about taking notes just yet, I'm going to list our favorite grocery items later in the book. True Lemon and True Lime come in a variety of flavors, but those are our personal favorites. They're simply packets of flavored powders, and they come in larger sizes for making pitchers as well as small packets for flavoring individual glasses or bottles of water. They're great to put in your purse for when you're going out and you're just not in the mood for water or iced tea.

It took way less time than I thought for all of us to completely abandon our favorite drinks in favor of healthier options; my kids were reaching for the healthy stuff without any complaint. I was continuing to see radical changes in my kids just from a protein-centered breakfast, reducing sugar/artificial sweetener consumption, and a major increase in water intake. Major changes were happening just from a few small adjustments. I was thrilled!

I'm sure there are a few people out there who are outraged that my kids were drinking soda or eating white toast and cereal in the first place. Hey, I knew then that those things weren't great for us, but I also know our conveniently packaged American lifestyle is really hard to fight. We're a very busy family: Jack and I work all the time, our kids each have busy schedules, and we have a farm that requires constant attention and work. We're not the only busy family, either. Most families have one, if not two, parents working a minimum of forty hours a week, plus after school activities for kids, church commitments, sports… the list is endless. Which makes it all too easy to just pick the easiest, quickest food option, even if we know, intellectually, it isn't the best choice.

I think that for many of us, especially working mothers, food and nutrition can take a back seat to the host of other things on our proverbial plate. Just yesterday I was at the dance studio with my daughter watching a mom run in with McDonalds for her daughter to eat between classes. It's not ideal, but guess what? It happens. And I'm certainly not one to judge because I've done it, too. Haven't we all?

But here's the thing: I really, truly believe that so many of the physical, emotional, and mental issues we're seeing in our kids are caused by poor nutrition. Here's just one example: My oldest son is wonderful, handsome, inspiring…and he's also on the autism spectrum. He's very high functioning, so most people would never even be able to tell without having personal experience themselves with high-functioning autistics. In just a few months on our adjusted diet, my son's grades went up, his sleep habits improved, his fidgeting lessened, and he was able to stop taking his medications on the weekends. He lost weight because he started running regularly with us; he's completed several five-kilometer runs now and he's always the one who finishes first—this is a child who just a few short months ago couldn't run a mile without stopping.

Having shared this, I have to say that I don't think my family is that uncommon. My kids are not the exceptions.

I think changing what we eat might even be easier than we think. I believe we've made this hard on ourselves. The collective "we" I'm speaking of here isn't just the average person, but also the food industry, and the diet-and-exercise industry, too. Whoever "we" is, whoever decided this is how we should eat and how we should live, is about to be challenged by me. I'm going to use my children, my life, and my home as an example. We'll be a case study.

As scary as that statement is for me, I feel it's my duty to lay it out there for you. I'm actually a very private person—surprising right?

I just keep thinking that if I can help one family, one mother, one child who's struggling with weight and health issues, I know it'll be worth it. Just stay with me. I've got so much to say and so many more examples to give. We can do this!

Once my family had eliminated our major food crutches, I started thinking maybe this was a little *too* easy. Why was I taking baby steps with this? I was seeing such amazing results—none of the kids were crying about eating more veggies (notice I'm not mentioning Jack), and we were all looking and feeling so much healthier. Even our skin was clearer. I mean, really, this was going pretty darn well.

So, naturally, I decided to jump straight off the cliff—I grabbed some trash bags and entered my pantry. I should mention we are very blessed to have an amazing pantry in our home. With so many kids, one of the major features of our house is an amazing kitchen with a walk-in butler's pantry, which is seriously a *dream* for a mom of six. We had a lot of food in that pantry which, I was realizing, was not the best or healthiest choices for us. So, I gave it all away. Every single last cereal box, granola bar, and packet of fruit snacks, even the Cheez-Its! It was all gone, and it felt both scary and awesome at the same time. I still wasn't exactly sure at that point what we *were* going to eat, but I knew it wouldn't be any of that crap.

Then I did something extreme: I ordered every cookbook in the Amazon Top One Hundred. Yes, it cost me a small fortune, but my family's health was worth it.

I had more studying to do. (More on that later).

My kids were already telling me how they were trying to make the healthiest choices they could at lunch. A few of them had even talked to their teachers and the school lunch providers about the sugar in the snacks and lunches they were eating. I was so proud of how proactive they were being! I never pushed them or told them what they could or couldn't eat; we just discussed the nutritional values of different food items, and we told them to always try to make the best choice at each meal.

I never wanted them to feel the pressure of making food choices that were off limits or wrong, because I knew from long, painful personal experience how demoralizing that can be. I didn't want them to walk around feeling guilty or ashamed if they had a bagel or a slice of pizza now and then. I just wanted them to be informed. I wanted them to see the results of good nutrition, and the changes in their bodies when they made healthy choices. Heck, that's what I wanted for myself! I just wanted to see our whole family reap the rewards of being as healthy as we could.

Which gave me another great idea that both scared me and excited me: I wanted us all to start running together. I was sure I could get the kids on board.

I just had to convince Jack.

Chapter 8

MOM FIGURES IT OUT:
SUGAR IS THE ENEMY, FATS ARE YOUR FRIEND

So back when I was a kid you'll remember I was told *ad nauseam* that fat was bad. Fat was the enemy. Fat was horrible. Don't ever eat Fat. This was so ingrained in my head that, without even thinking, I always grabbed whatever product was labeled "fat free" at the grocery store. It made me a fatty-food bigot and, as an adult, I still carried that bias. But as I was investigating different diet books and health plans and reading scientific studies, I was quickly realizing that all the understanding regarding fat and its effects had changed.

Fat wasn't what was made me fat—it was all the sugar.

The collective wisdom from decades of scientific study is that some fat in your diet is okay, and even necessary. Fats just aren't as bad for you as we once thought them to be, and they're certainly not the be-all and end-all cause of obesity.

My number one goal is to make this book as easy to understand and helpful as possible, because after reading the top one hundred health and diet books, my head was spinning. Most of them are completely contradictory and over half weren't at all family-friendly.

I kept thinking how hard it was to wade through the vast amount information that's out there. I won't share all of the science behind my plan, but please know everything I'm telling you is based on both science and research. You can find this research for yourself if you're interested. I am lucky I'm both a speed-reader and a person who likes to consider all the information available before making a decision about which way to go. I'm a studier, and I never do what people tell me—my husband says it's both a blessing and a curse to be married to such a hardheaded woman.

All of my reading was making me angry. Why is it so hard for us to get healthy? Why are there so many gimmicks and unnecessary costs associated with being healthy? Why is health so damn hard for us as Americans? I think a huge part of it is that there are just too many people looking to make a quick buck, and too many people desperate to lose weight, which has lead to this constant stream of next "hot diets" or "easy weight loss systems."

What follows is the truth I've gleaned from all those contradictory studies and how, as a result of a lot of trial and error, it has worked for my family and me.

Every other diet book is going to tell you that carbs are bad for you. Paleo, Ketogenic, and Atkins all have their place on the top 100 health charts. But let me tell you why I still eat healthy carbs—note the phrasing, it's an important distinction: *healthy carbs*. First, I've lost a lot of weight while still eating them and second, I don't think that eliminating any of the God-created food groups is necessary or healthy. If you have a legitimate, food-specific allergy, then that's a whole different story. One of my very best friends has Celiac Disease and I'm not going to debate food elimination in those cases; it's necessary and non-negotiable.

But in the case of carbs, especially when it comes to feeding my children, it's best not to throw out the baby with the bathwater. I think the way companies process grains is harmful to us, but whole, unprocessed foods like oats, flax, sweet potatoes, quinoa, brown rice, and breads made from sprouted grains are both healthy and necessary, and can actually aid in weight loss.

Again, this is contradictory to most of the books I read, but I want you to know about *my* personal experience. I believe carbs are very important for kids, because they give them energy and aid growth. My kids love to add some rice to their dinner, or start off the day with old-fashioned oats with some yogurt and berries mixed in.

One of the main reasons I think so many of us have failed diet after diet is that it becomes unmaintainable in the long-term. We lose those last few pounds and then we go right back to business as usual. And then guess what happens?

Vrrrroooooooot! Our weight balloons right back up to where we were, if not even higher. Right? I know you've experienced it, too.

So when I set out to create a whole new system of healthy eating for my family, I knew we needed to make it something we could all live with long-term. I didn't want anyone to feel deprived; I wanted us to be excited about the food we ate. I also wanted them to have a voice in what we decided to eat, and why. My older three kids now read the labels even when they're at school; I started getting emails from teachers telling me they heard my kids questioning some of the snacks they were offered at school, and suggesting healthier alternatives…and their peers and the school staff were listening! This was honestly surprising to me—my kids were taking their nutrition seriously, all on their own! It blew my mind.

As time went on, and my family continued to feel better and look better, I decided to be a bit bolder in what I asked of them. On

Halloween we decided we would still go trick or treating, but we would donate our candy. We dressed up in our costumes and went downtown to see all the fun costumes and to take part in the annual parade. Then we went home and I made them special treats: sugar-free donuts, flavored popcorn, and dark chocolate.

I'm sure there are people out there rolling their eyes and shouting about how I ruined Halloween, so let me give you another reason to write me angry emails. We all ran a 5k race that day, and here's the crazy thing: my kids said it was the best Halloween they'd ever had. They loved the 5k and the special treats I had made, and no one, not even the three and four year-olds, asked for sugary candy. They didn't even miss it!

How crazy is that?

I think we often underestimate our kids—I know I do. I also know it's sometimes hard to find a good balance between when to really push them on something and when to just let them coast. I think in terms of nutrition and health we always need to push. We need to help them understand the importance of being in control of what goes into their bodies, especially when they are preteens as my older three are. Become informed, mama. Tell them *why* certain things aren't a great choice and see what they do on their own. Above all, if you are a good example, your kids will rise to the occasion, too.

I've listed below what we *don't* eat because it's a much shorter list than what we *do* eat. Also, I've given you some great resources for finding family-friendly recipes that your husband and kids will *rave* about (Pinterest is your friend). We never focus on weight in my family; our conversations are about health, how we feel, our strength, and our energy levels. Yes, there are very noticeable physical differences in my family that I want to share with you, but our number one goal has been and always will be health and wellness.

Strong is the new sexy; healthy is the new black.
Being healthy is the new American dream!

FOODS WE AVOID, AND WHAT WE BUY INSTEAD:

- **No to sugar.** Yes, all sugar. Did you know sugar is also the main cause of heart disease? Get rid of the sugar! Be aware that many packaged foods contain sugar, ketchup for example. Read the labels and try to choose something different. We use natural Stevia instead, and sometimes xylitol or erythritol. If you use xylitol be careful that your dog doesn't get it, as it can be lethal to them. My kids LOVE True Lemon and True Lime sweeteners. You can buy them at your local store and they are usually found near the powdered, packaged drinks.

- **No to most cereals and granola.** We substitute these with the Ezekiel and Uncle Sam brands which we love. We often add them to our yogurt for some crunch. A little goes a long way!

- **No to anything you would get from a bakery.** Yes, even cupcakes…especially cupcakes!

- **No to whole-wheat pasta.** Instead, we eat brown rice and Dreamfields pasta in place of regular pasta. Dreamfields is especially good for replacing that macaroni and cheese your little ones insist on.

- **No to regular bread**—white or wheat, or even "whole wheat". My family eats only Ezekiel and/or other sprouted grain breads. You can find them in the freezer section of your grocery market, and my local Target even has a brand that is kid-approved.

- **No to all the "normal" American snack foods.** We don't do granola bars, crackers, cookies, chips, or pretzels. My kids do like to snack, so it was important to find good substitutions. One of our favorites is WASA crackers; we do so much with these! They're a low glycemic, low sugar cracker which we slather liberally with Laughing Cow cheese, cream cheese, or natural peanut butter and low sugar jelly for a PB+J snack. My kids like them topped with almost anything, even cucumbers. I will say that the longer they've been off sugar the better they like them. We also add them to soups and chili. My kids also *love* nuts! I try to keep a tray out in the kitchen at all times filled with almonds, pistachios, and cashews, which all have good healthy fats and proteins that will help curb hunger. Nuts and veggies are sometimes a bit more expensive, but we try to shop local and use lots of farmers markets and farm stands. If you are able to access those, it can mean great savings on your food bill. Your health is worth it!

- **No to ice cream, sorbet, popsicles, and yogurt with added sugar.** This can be difficult for kids, and parents too. The great thing is that we live in a day and age where there are lots of alternatives. I took my kids shopping with me and we found some things that they liked that were good for them. We all eat Bryers Carb Smart Ice Cream topped with some Fat Free Reddi Whip, or a few Lily's stevia-sweetened chocolate chips. Yes, those chocolate chips are expensive but it's worth it. Because you only need a few, a package can last a long time. We also indulge in Halo Top brand ice cream for very special occasions. We also make our own shakes with fresh berries, almond milk, ice, yogurt, and stevia. Jack and I often add whey protein powder to a shake after we've done a run or a workout. We only use Greek yogurt, mostly the Oikos Triple Zero brand as they have great flavors my family loves. When it goes on sale we often buy out the store's entire supply—if you ask, some stores will even sell you the wholesale box they received. Just as an FYI, the banana flavor is wonderful to use for making pancakes. And now I'm hungry.

- **No to soda and juice.** We don't drink soda or juice, as I've already mentioned. Did you know one can of soda per day increases a child's risk of becoming obese by 60 percent? *One* can. Our drinks of choice are mostly sparkling water and tea. Other great options are Zevia, Honest Fizz, and Blue Sky Zero. These are all pop alternatives sweetened with Stevia. They're basically sparkling water, but they have a sweeter taste, and they have great flavor choices—we're huge fans of the Vanilla Cherry Crème from Blue Sky Zero, which you can find on Amazon. Jack and I also drink the occasional light beer or dry red wine. I know that's also contrary to many current health and diet ideas out there, but I think wine has many health benefits (more on that later).

- **No to anything that has a ton of unpronounceable ingredients.** If we do buy prepackaged foods, we make sure they have a minimal list of ingredients; if we can't pronounce it and the list is more than five or so items long, we probably won't eat it. Yes, we do make exceptions, but that's our general rule. Don't eat something if you can't figure out what's in it. Eat as many natural, God made, whole foods as possible. Fresh is best!

FOOD MY FAMILY LOVES:
- Oikos Triple Zero yogurt.

- Ezekiel brand breads and cereals—they even have English muffins for making a little pizza or breakfast sandwich!
- WASA brand crackers
- Berries, fresh and frozen
- Eggs—farm fresh are the best!
- Applegate brand sausages (OMG, so good)
- Pancakes made from oats
- Veggies—eat them in season to save money. Local farmers markets are awesome.
- Lily's brand chocolate and Dr. John's candy (Ahhh-mazing)
- Dreamfields pasta
- Meat and seafood—we try to do local and grass-fed when we can. Laura's Beef at our local store often goes on sale and I stock up when it does.
- Almond milk—we love Califia Farms brand
- Fairlife brand milk
- Breyer's Carb Smart ice cream (yes, this has a bit of Splenda in it, but not enough that I'm going to lose sleep over it.)
- Nuts—my family loves nuts, especially almonds and cashews
- Baked blue corn chips
- Mission brand low carb wraps (we use these for roll-ups in place of sandwiches, and for "Taco Tuesday", and for lots of other things listed at the end of the book)
- Kerry's Gold brand butter—yep, the real stuff
- Sour cream
- Cheese—the real stuff, nothing processed or fake
- Oils—I use mostly coconut oil and olive oil
- Lots of herbs and spices. Don't think your kids won't like them. My kids have really grown to want everything seasoned.

- Simple Girl BBQ sauce (can be found at Amazon)
- Quest brand protein bars—great after a run or a workout
- Jay Robb brand and Quest brand protein powders. Again, great after a workout
- Lesser Evil brand popcorn—found on Amazon (be careful, that stuff is addictive!)
- Bai 5 brand drinks
- Vitamin Water Zero

Most of these items *are* more expensive than their counterparts. It's stupid and it sucks, but nothing is more important than your health. I'm a bargain shopper ninja, so I shop sales and stock up in mass quantity whenever I can. When our local co-op puts Lily's chocolate bars on sale I've been known to buy them in embarrassing quantity, but my family *loves* them for treats and, hey, half-off is half-off. When you find things you know your family loves, keep an eye out for when the prices go down and stock up big time. Some stores will give you a nice discount if you buy in bulk quantities, so ask!

Will what worked for my family work for you exactly the same way? Probably not, but I think making the healthiest choices you can for your family is vitally important. I believe the diseases plaguing our kids, and us as adults, at increasingly high rates, are intrinsically related to what we put inside our bodies, often without thinking about it. So start thinking! Read the ingredients. Look and see if you recognize the things in the ingredient list of the foods you buy.

Below is the ingredient list, taken from Wikipedia, for a popular breakfast product. Do you know which cereal it is?

"Oats (Whole grain), Oats (flour), marshmallows (sugar, modified starch/modified corn starch, corn syrup, dextrose, gelatin, calcium carbonate, yellow 5 & yellow 6, blue 1, red 40), artificial flavor, sugar,

corn syrup, corn starch, salt, calcium carbonate, food coloring/artificial color, trisodium phosphate, zinc, iron, vitamin C (sodium ascorbic), niacinamide (a B vitamin), vitamin B2 (riboflavin), vitamin B1 (thiamin mononitrate), vitamin A (palmitate), folic acid, vitamin B12, vitamin D, vitamin E (mixed tocopherols)."

What the hell is niacinamide? Palmitate? Thiamin mononitrate?

Do you recognize that product? It's Lucky Charms. The manufacturers say those things are "vitamins", but why do you need to add them in the first place? Fresh whole foods have all the vitamins and minerals you'll ever need.

Pro tip: if you can't find some of these recommended items in your local store, check Amazon—they almost always have them in stock and some are even available for auto delivery, bulk quantity, or pantry boxes for an even better discount. You can also use the website "store locator" for hard-to-find items. Asking your grocery store to order them for you might also be an option; mine gives a discount for special bulk orders.

Chapter 9:

KEEPING IT SIMPLE: LET'S START IN THE KITCHEN

MY HUSBAND AND CHILDREN DON'T REALLY NEED TO SHED any weight, as they've all reached a place where they're within the normal range for their height and age. Two of my children lost about ten pounds each that had them close to an unhealthy weight according to their doctor. This weight loss was due to the changes we had made in terms of food intake and activity levels. My other kids had issues that were not at all connected to weight, and these all improved once we changed our diet. They've since maintained their new, healthier weights, and our doctor is pleased with their overall health progress.

My weight had always been at the root of my long laundry list of health problems and I felt I was basically becoming carbohydrate-intolerant. Virtually any sugar made me feel yucky, my blood disorder and the lack of nutrients in my blood was also causing some issues.

I believe that balancing your blood sugar levels is key to your overall health and I knew I'd have to start managing my blood sugar and insulin levels. At this point, I decided to include several superfoods to my diet (see the list of superfoods in Chapter 11), as well as some additional vitamin supplements. I also read a handful of books on the concept of food cycling, and I immediately decided that it made sense and I wanted to try it.

In a nutshell, food cycling is eating certain foods together at the same time and cycling carbs in and out of your diet, so that you can burn off body fat more easily. There are several different ways to do this, and I found lots of contradictory information on the subject. Some books suggested eating carbs one week and not eating them the next, while other books recommended having carbs with every other meal, and still others said to rotate a few days on and a few days off.

Needless to say, all this new information seemed very complicated, and the rules were very confusing to me, so I set out to come up with a plan that would be easy for me and my busy schedule. And…I had to create meal plans that would accommodate my eating preferences with those of my family members.

My solution? I let my family lead the way. I knew from my research that I wanted to try and keep healthy, carb-friendly meals separate from meals with fats, so I would plan meals for my entire family and then structure my specific plan around that. What does that look like? Well, if my family has Taco Tuesday with low carb Mission wraps, I'm going to skip the cheese and do a low fat sour cream or tacos on lettuce wraps. Sometimes I'll have oatmeal for breakfast three or four days in a row, and then when my whole family decides they want omelets I'll join them, and add some turkey bacon or chicken sausage. My kids will usually add toast with some low sugar jelly.

For lunch Jack and I almost always eat a chef's salad. It is loaded with protein and it fills us up for the whole afternoon. My go to snack is yogurt—I *love* yogurt, and sometimes I'll add some Ezekiel cereal for crunch in the morning, or mix in a few chocolate chips and freeze it for a bedtime snack. It's actually really funny because as much as I love yogurt, Jack hates it. He won't even touch the container. He says he has some repressed childhood memories. He's so weird. ;-)

I do track my calories with a fitness app just so I'm sure I'm staying within range, and I don't go crazy with any one particular food group. Protein and greens are daily staples, and I try to make sure I'm always getting enough fluids. Drinking all day is tough, though, because I have to pee all day, but I've also come to realize I'm often dehydrated, which can cause false hunger, so make sure you're drinking enough. Tea—both iced and hot—is what I try to go for during the day. We have a whole cupboard containing many different types of tea. Jack and I both keep a big thermos of hot tea on our desk, so we keep drinking throughout the day. I'm sure you can find some sort of tea you like—I've seen everything from watermelon tea to chocolate tea. It's great for your body, too!

As far as developing family recipes of our own, I've found a few great cookbooks we use on a regular basis, and we also use Pinterest a lot—we have a Pinterest board only we can see and we pin things we think the family might like. My amazing nanny helps with meal planning and shopping, and we often modify recipes that have things we are trying to stay away from, substituting the bad ingredient for something healthier. If you find a sweetener you really like—we love Swerve brand—you can just use that if the recipe calls for sugar. I even came up with a corn casserole modification for Thanksgiving that my kids thought was decent.

There *is* a bit of a learning curve to all this, but there are amazing bloggers, vloggers, and moms out there working on family-approved, low-sugar, low- or no-carb meals. Be confident, you can do it.

Let's just be honest for a minute, here: I'm a mom of six, a bestselling author, and I run a 50-acre farm—I don't have the time to make gourmet meals for my kids. The few recipes of my own I'm including in this book come from a busy woman who just wants to give her kids healthy foods they'll actually eat, enjoy, and gain nourishment from. If you're looking for fancy, you won't find it here.

GET READY AND STOCK UP!

I've included a list of things that are great to have in your pantry, and I bet you have many of these things in your kitchen already. These are my regular go-to utensils and products. But, please, let me say it is not necessary to run out and buy everything to start with. Just add these things gradually as you go.

Let me say again that your health is an important investment. Fresh ingredients make good foods; they will always taste better than things that come in a package.

Let food be thy medicine and medicine be thy food. – Hippocrates

KITCHEN UTENSILS:
- A good set of knives
- A good set of pans (these don't have to be expensive). I really like the Stone Earth pans by Ozeri. Stainless steel or cast iron are also both great choices.
- Stainless steel measuring cups and spoons
- A nice 9-inch ceramic baking dish—I have an enameled cast iron dish by Cuisinart and I love it!
- A large skillet
- Nice, sturdy mixing bowls
- A good blender. Ninja, Vitamix, or Blendtec are all great. But a blender doesn't have to be new or top of the line to get the job done; my mom still uses the one she bought in the 70s.
- I love a good wok for preparing stir-frys. Meat, veggies,

some coconut oil, and spices make a quick and yummy dinner.

- I also love the new multi-cookers, a newer take on a regular old crockpot. If you haven't seen those yet, check them out. They make cooking so much faster and easier, and busy moms always need more convenience, right?

- A few pretty plates and mugs are always nice to have—don't save all the nice dinnerware for holidays! We eat our morning omelets on really cute Pioneer Woman plates I got at Walmart. I always feel special in the morning when we use them. There is a truth to the saying that "we eat with our eyes"—make every meal a reason to get out the good dishes. Fueling your body is important so, take your time, enjoy the process, and make it pretty!

FOR YOUR PANTRY:

- Old-fashioned oats—I use these for so many things!
- WASA crackers are so versatile! Use them with Laughing Cow cheese, veggies, berries, and even chocolate!
- Nuts, nut butters, and nut flours
- Brown rice
- Quinoa
- Coconut oil. This oil is amazing! Pour it in your mouth, on your skin, and all over your food. Honestly, where has coconut oil been all my life? It's ahhhh-mazing!
- Extra virgin olive oil (for low and medium temperature cooking only)
- Spices—my favorites are ginger, cinnamon, cayenne pepper, pink sea salt (pink sea salt is wonderful for you. We buy it in bulk on Amazon. Amazing health benefits!),

pepper, chili powder, oregano, garlic, turmeric, and basil
- Sugar and chemical-free protein powder
- Mustard
- Apple cider vinegar—add this to your LaCroix sparkling water with some True Lemon. This is a tasty combo, sweet like soda but good for you; the health benefits of apple cinder vinegar are listed in the supplements section.
- Sugar-free pasta sauce; we *love* the Classico Riserva
- Dark chocolate (70% cocao or higher), or stevia sweetened
- Pyure or Swerve stevia
- Seeds such as hemp, chia, buckwheat
- Cocoa powder
- Coffee and tea
- LaCroix sparkling water
- True Lemon or True Lime

FOR YOUR FRIDGE:
- Power greens such as kale, Swiss chard, spinach, dark green lettuce. Salads are wonderful for lunch.
- Eggs—give us this day our daily eggs! These are the perfect food; so don't leave them out of your diet!
- Almond milk
- Cream cheese
- Oikos Triple Zero Greek yogurt
- Sour cream
- Cottage cheese
- All non-processed cheeses
- Mayonnaise (we really like the Just Mayo brand)

- Real butter
- Veggies
- Fresh salsa
- Lots of low sugar fruits: lemons, limes, and berries are great for infusing into your water.
- Meat—I prefer to eat meat that is still on the bone. It has nutrients that boneless cuts do not have. Get some wings, thighs, and even whole chickens. My kids *love* wing night and we feel really wild and primal ripping that juicy meat off the bone.

FOR YOUR FREEZER:

- Meats of all kinds—it's really your choice. We stock up when things go on sale. Check your SAM's Club and Costco for good prices on organic meat. My freezer is currently full of grass-fed beef because I saw it for a steal of a deal at Meijer. Wait for a sale and buy all you can; healthy doesn't have to mean expensive. Also, you will eat less of the good stuff. Good organic meat does not have added fillers, and it allows you to stay full longer.
- I *always* keep frozen berries to add to smoothies and our morning oatmeal mush.
- Spinach is always great to keep frozen. Spinach is loaded in protein and iron and you won't even taste it in your smoothie—even Jack adds it to his post-workout smoothies, and I told you how he feels about veggies.
- We also buy sprouted-grain bread and keep that in our freezer. Yes, these are expensive but I also buy in bulk when I see a good sale price.
- Frozen organic veggies (often cheaper than the fresh, but

still good)

FRUIT AND SUGAR:

Yes, fruit has natural sugars, but some affect your body more than others. I'm not okay with cutting all fruit from your diet, because I believe God gave us these tasty treats for a reason. Just know that some fruits are going to be better and easier on your body than others. Below is a list of fruits that include the best and the worst at keeping your insulin levels in a good place. And remember: all things in moderation.

- The best fruits: blueberries, raspberries, lemons, limes, avocado and tomatoes. Two servings per day of these is fine.
- Okay-but-not-great fruits: green apples, kiwi, grapefruit, honeydew melon, mandarins, plums, peaches, pears, nectarines, strawberries and oranges. If you do choose these fruits try to limit them to one per day.
- On occasion fruits: grapes, cherries, red apples, pineapple, papaya, mangoes, and bananas. Because of the high fructose levels in these fruits they should be eaten very rarely.

BE CHOOSY WITH YOUR GRAINS:

Not all grains or carbohydrates have been created equally; some have a very negative impact on your body, and others are good for you. Most people are aware that things like regular factory-processed bread, cakes, cereals, cookies, and crackers are bad for you, but did you know barley and rye could have similar damaging affects on your body?

- The best grains: buckwheat, millet, oats, quinoa, brown

rice and flax

- Sprouted breads are always the best choice. You find these in the freezer section of your grocery store.

Pro tip: Shop the perimeter of your grocery store: they usually put all the food you don't want front and center by the entrances, and in the middle! Also, eating a protein bar before you shop will help you avoid making impulse purchases—shopping when we're hungry can be dangerous! Stalk the sales, and buy in bulk! If you keep your pantry stocked with all the good stuff you will be less inclined to go for that no-no on the back shelf. Also, really examine the ingredients lists for things like salad dressing, pasta sauce, peanut butter and flavored water, because they often include sugar.

Chapter 10

MY DIVORCE FROM SUGAR; DETOX IS HELL

"One cannot think well, love well, sleep well,
if one has not dined well."
— Virginia Woolf

I RECENTLY READ THAT THE AVERAGE AMERICAN EATS OVER A hundred and fifty *pounds* of sugar each year, *triple* what we consumed just a hundred years ago. That sort of increase is causing not just obesity, but all the related illnesses that come along with it.

Sometimes it is hard to avoid sugar altogether. It's amazing how many different foods have a high sugar content; start looking, and you'll see what I mean. Sugar is in *everything*! If the second ingredient is sugar, put it down and walk away.

THE MANY NAMES FOR SUGAR:
- Agave nectar
- Barbados sugar
- Barley malt
- Barley malt syrup
- Beet sugar

- Brown sugar
- Buttered syrup
- Cane juice
- Cane juice crystals
- Cane sugar
- Caramel
- Carob syrup
- Castor sugar
- Coconut palm sugar
- Coconut sugar
- Confectioner's sugar
- Corn sweetener
- Corn syrup
- Corn syrup solids
- Date sugar
- Dehydrated cane juice
- Demerara sugar
- Dextrin
- Dextrose
- Evaporated cane juice
- Free-flowing brown sugars
- Fructose
- Fruit juice
- Fruit juice concentrate
- Glucose
- Glucose solids
- Golden sugar
- Golden syrup
- Grape sugar
- HFCS (High-Fructose Corn Syrup)

- Honey
- Icing sugar
- Invert sugar
- Malt syrup
- Maltodextrin
- Maltol
- Maltose
- Mannose
- Maple syrup
- Molasses
- Muscovado
- Palm sugar
- Panocha
- Powdered sugar
- Raw sugar
- Refiner's syrup
- Rice syrup
- Saccharose
- Sorghum Syrup
- Sucrose
- Sugar (granulated)
- Sweet Sorghum
- Syrup
- Treacle
- Turbinado sugar
- Yellow sugar

Detox from sugar can be actual hell. The average American is addicted to both sugar and carbs, and it's a very hard addiction to break. You can experience flu-like symptoms. You might even question your sanity. And it may take days or even weeks to kick the addiction.

Here's why: sugar is a drug.

For many of us, even if we refuse to admit it, sugar has a hold on us and, in my case, a near-fatal hold.

Before my last pregnancy and my detox from sugar, I would crave things *so* badly—I would lose focus just *thinking* about a sweet treat. I would often go out of my way just to pass the bakery. This is not just a "fat kid" thing, this is more normal than abnormal, I think. I could see the same thing happening to my kids, and I could really see it in my borderline-diabetic husband. His cravings and low and high sugar spikes turned him into another person. He would be irritable, sleepy, and angry from the sugar rollercoaster.

If there is one piece of advice you take away from this book, it needs to be this: CUT OUT THE SUGAR. It's nasty stuff. Elevated blood sugar levels are now known to be toxic to the brain. I truly believe the increase in neurological disorders in our country is directly linked to the food we are eating. Things like ADHD, depression, chronic headache, insomnia, autism, anxiety, epilepsy and schizophrenia have all been directly correlated to diet.

Our bodies are just not equipped to handle these kinds of foods and in the quantity we as a culture are consuming them. People are eating too many processed foods, foods that are virtually devoid of any nutrients and that are jammed full of chemicals.

Cute little things like animal crackers, pure sugar shaped into little fruits, cereals liberally sprinkled with marshmallows, and ultra-processed grains shaped into flakes literally *coated* in frosting… these kinds of things are seriously harming our children.

They're not just *bad* for us, they're *killing* us.

It seems every new scientific study reveals another illness caused by poor nutrition. Even cancer has been directly linked to diet! But don't just take my word for it—I'm not a doctor, I'm just an angry mom. Please read *Always Hungry* by Dr. David Ludwig, *Grain Brain* by Dr. David Perlmutter, or watch the Internet video *The Skinny on Obesity* by the University of California with Dr. Robert Lustig.

Please become aware of the crap we are being fed—and I mean that literally—in terms of the way the effects of highly processed, high caloric and low nutrient foods are being downplayed. I believe these kinds of foods are harmful at worst, and are doing nothing good for us at best. I believe we need to take a stand and demand that the food industry make changes, and start giving us more options. We've reached epidemic levels when it comes to the number of people affected by metabolic syndromes—currently over 60% of all Americans are affected by a metabolic syndrome of some kind.

How many people do you know with heart disease, hypertension, type 2 diabetes, dementia, cancer, PCOS or liver disease? How many kids do you know with ADD or ADHD? We now have scientific studies that make a direct correlation between these things and what we're eating.

Is it any wonder we are seeing such an increase in neurological disorders, seeing that our culture is consuming *more* sugar each year?

Once my family broke free from sugar and were past the detox phase, we honestly began to feel like different people. We had crazy energy, and I'm not talking about something like a sugar-high or a caffeine-buzz energy spurt—this new sugar-free energy is constant and steady. We don't have the afternoon crash. We feel stronger, and we sleep better, too. I can point to each one of my children and say they've had a dramatic change in their physical wellness just from consuming less sugar.

And, by the way, artificial sweeteners like aspartame count as sugar, and are even *worse* than sugar. So switching to "diet" soda doesn't count. Sorry! Those artificial sweeteners are awful for you, too.

Even though I have said previously that our way might not work for every family, I *do* firmly and passionately believe that cutting out sugar will make *everyone* feel better. It may take some adjustment, there will be a detox phase, and it might take weeks or months, but it *will* be worth it.

My dear father came to visit us when we were just beginning to make these changes. After eating the dinner I'd made, he told me it tasted like wood. If you know my dad, then you know that comment was actually pretty kind. But then, this past Christmas, when he was up visiting I made a cheesecake he raved about, and he wanted more to take home. What he didn't know was that I had sent my mother some of the stevia sweetener I use, and she'd been using it in her cooking and baking as well, and he didn't even realize it! This is just further proof that, yes, it does sometimes require baby steps to make changes.

Baby steps are *fine*! None of us got healthy in a single day, or with a single meal. The journey to becoming strong and healthy can take some time. Give yourself that time and grace. Don't give up. Keep moving forward—you're worth it!

Life without sugar can look weird to some people. Some of my friends poke fun at my family. I'm often seen passing out True Lemon packets to my kids when we're out to eat. I'm the mom that packs Ziploc bags of nuts and handfuls of Quest bars in my purse. I've been known to send my kids to school with a snack of colorful sliced bell peppers. Hey, it's cool to be weird, right?

I think that for many of you reading, this all sounds a little crazy.

If you had told me a year ago that I would lose over 100 pounds—again—and write a family health book, I would have laughed at you…but crazier things have happened. It's okay to do this your way. It's okay for your family to find things that work for you and you alone.

For example, my family doesn't really like avocado. I'm sure many of you want to throw this book across the room just because of that fact alone, but we really don't. We've tried. I know there are many awesome things that can be done with avocado and I hope your family adopts them as new favorites.

This book isn't a one size fits all. But it is about what it takes for your family to be healthy and strong. What does health look like to you? Just take that first step to find out.

QUICK AND EASY TIPS FOR CUTTING OUT SUGAR:
- Start with one meal at a time—breakfast first
- Don't dump your whole pantry if that doesn't work for you or your budget; slowly make changes in the things you buy, phase things out. This isn't all-or-nothing—look at the big picture.
- What are your go-to staples? Do you love popcorn and wine at night? What's the healthiest way to do that? Maybe change the sugary, sweet wine for something dry and red? How about a Skinny Girl 100 pack of popcorn instead of the butter flavor you usually buy?
- Increase your water intake. This is a detox, so we need to flush this junk out. Make sure you stay hydrated. Not to be gross, but pee shouldn't be bright yellow or orange, and it shouldn't smell super pungent. If it does look and smell like this, then you are dehydrated.
- Focus on your proteins. I make my kids do something I call

the "meat challenge." It's just a fun game for them to try and eat all of their protein first. At each meal they try to eat all the protein first and then go to the other things on the plate: this is the meat challenge. We've found that protein fills them up and keeps them that way—which means they snack less, we spend less on snacks and we eat better foods as a result! This has been wonderful for my two younger sons who always get excited when they complete the "meat challenge." We make it a big deal for them. Before our dietary changes, they would sometimes refuse to eat the main course or maybe even dinner itself. Now, they are eating healthy at every meal. It's really wonderful for me to see everyone satisfied at each meal. I can't tell you how stressful it was when my kids didn't want to eat for whatever reason. I think it was often because they "craved" bread and sugar. Now that they are off the sugar, I'm seeing them eat a variety of foods that I wouldn't have imagined possible before.

The great thing about detox is that it doesn't last forever. It might be rough for a few days or weeks, but once you've come out of the sugar-fog you'll feel like a million bucks! My sugar detox wasn't as bad as some I've read about, as I didn't get crazy headaches or feel achy all over. If anything, I just felt "weird." I did immediately feel a change in my body, though—it really felt like someone had flipped a switch. I'm not really sure why, because I've tried cutting out sugar before. I think my resistance was just better this time. I didn't have an urge to cheat at all. Once I had passed a certain point, sugar didn't even look appetizing anymore.

Jack and I were at a signing right after the baby was born, and a reader brought some of the best looking cupcakes I had ever seen from a fancy bakery in New York. The smell was intoxicating and they were a work of art. Did I eat one? Nope, sure didn't. I really wasn't even tempted. I had my Lily's chocolate bar in my purse and I was going to have it as a treat once we were done. I ended up giving the cupcakes away and I know they were thoroughly enjoyed. Would I have beat myself up had I had some? No. But I just didn't *want* them. I made a choice and I was proud of myself.

The food choices I made on that trip were so shocking to my mother that it started her on her own health journey. Now, at age sixty-five, she's also down several pounds, feeling better, and recovering from the chronic stomach pain and irritable bowl syndrome she's struggled with for many years. Until she tried my plan, she hadn't been able to lose any weight at all in fifteen years! I don't think age or stage of life play any part in this, either. If my three year-old and my mother can see amazing results just from cutting out sugar, you can too! I would love to see mothers, daughters and grandmothers all doing this together. We need to encourage and inspire the best health for the ones we love. It's so important.

If sugar has been a friend to you like it's been to me, then this stage might be emotional. It's okay to miss your friends and it's okay to grieve. I'm not even being funny about this. Breaking up with my favorite foods was hard. Cupcakes were like a BFF to me, but I found other things that satisfied me even more.

Cheesecake and cookie bars are two of my most favorite holiday treats, and I was able to find two amazing recipes that surpassed my expectations this year. My kids loved it and raved that it was the best cheesecake they'd ever had. Did it take planning and time to find something I thought would take the place of our previous treats? Yes. Did it end up being a bit more costly to use the more expensive sweetener and sugar-free chocolate? Yes.

My family doesn't eat these sorts of treats on a daily basis, but for special occasions it's okay to go all out making treats everyone will enjoy. Life is about living, and being happy. Sharing a meal is part of that; especially when it comes to birthdays, holidays and other special days in the year so go all out! The best part will be that you won't feel sick or sluggish afterwards. No food comas! You will have energy to laugh and play together. Trust me on this!

Maybe there is a certain soda that you just can't live without, Diet Coke for example. I believe diet soda was a huge contributor to my weight gain and becoming bloated and inflamed. I was a Diet Sunkist addict for ten years, but I found an orange flavored Zevi that is a great replacement. Not as sweet, but it does the trick. The weird thing is that I don't even want that daily anymore. I have one maybe every few days when I think something would go well with it. But I'm not attached to it like I was with the Diet Sunkist drink. Surprising, but true.

Now, wine is a totally different story. You won't ever get me away from my wine. Please…bury me with a fancy bottle of Cabernet Sauvignon. Ha!

Honestly though, don't doubt your body's ability to roll with these changes.

One day at a time; you can do it! Start slow and don't go overboard. We want this to stick and we want it to work. If you want a lifestyle change to be sustainable, then it has to be able to be maintained long-term. Keep experimenting and find replacements for things containing sugar and I promise you it will continue to get better. If Jack can do it, you can do it. Just don't ask him to eat cauliflower…that's a hard limit for him.

Chapter 11

SEEING FOOD IN A WHOLE NEW WAY: FUEL VS. COMFORT

ABOUT THREE WEEKS INTO MAKING THESE HEALTHY CHANGES, your weight is going to go up, or you're going to get stressed out, or just hit a wall. It's bound to happen. Don't give up; you've got it!

My body chemistry and hormones were working in sync while I was pregnant with baby Ree, so the weight came off pretty easily and steadily, but after I had her my body was no longer with the plan. And, to this day, I'm not sure why. I just know my weight started to creep back up. There were a few days when I swore a lot and wanted to chuck my newly acquired scale out the window and then run it over with my truck a few times. Why the heck couldn't my body ever get with the freaking program? The more upset I got, the more I would use food as a comfort.

I was getting sucked right back into the old cycle.

I remember listening to Oprah talk about her battle with her weight and food, hearing her say she used food as a comfort as well. For me, though, I think the comfort was mostly out of habit; I knew my body didn't *need* the food to feel better, and I knew the food wouldn't even really make me feel better. In fact, the food usually just ended up making me feel worse. The issue was, comfort eating is what I always did, going back to my childhood when I would sneak snacks up to my room just because I was bored. There isn't really one specific thing I can point to as the single major contributor; it was just everything about Food, with a capital 'F'.

So what changed this time?

Well, I think I was finally at the point where I wanted to fight back, and fight *hard*. I was sick of the way I felt all the time. I hated the stigma of illness: asthma, bad knees, blood disorder, morbid obesity—my whole self, basically. I was finally at a point where I wasn't going to take it anymore. I knew there was no quick fix to this. There was no surgery, no pill, and no magic potion. This had to be a body, mind, and spirit change. I asked God to change my heart about food.

Now, I have to admit, I've been praying this prayer my whole life, but I just figured God was too busy with other stuff to deal with it. But, in all honesty, God *had* been giving me answers—I just didn't want to hear them.

This time, however, I felt like everything was laid out in front of me, obvious and undeniable.

First, I had to pick different foods. The ones God created, not man. Food that would nourish, heal, and fuel my body, not control it and drag me down. I also knew I had to get moving and get physically active.

That was it. I could see it as clear as day: healthy calories in, and constant physical movement.

It wasn't going to be easy, but that was the clear and direct answer from God Himself. Nothing in life worth having comes easy. That's been the theme of my life, and it might be yours, too. We have to want health over other things: over money, over time, over leisure. This isn't an easy pill to swallow, I know, but it's actually quite empowering.

I know there are going to be many times during the remainder of my life when I'm going to need comfort, when I'm going to need to be consoled, when I'm going to weep. I refuse to let food be the illusion of real comfort. Real comfort is my husband's arms, my friend's ear, or my child's laugh. Food will only mask or distract you from what you really and truly need. Don't give it that power over you. It's only fuel; you deserve real comfort.

POSTIVE SUBSTITUTIONS FOR COMFORT EATING:

- Sex—burns two hundred calories in thirty minutes when done correctly. Dude, that's a whole yogurt! Just sayin'.
- Exercise—I know it sounds crazy but you might actually grow to like it. I know I have!
- Turn on the music and dance. I've found some great YouTube videos featuring short dances set to my favorite songs. I've broken up my afternoon with one of those and felt so much better.
- Go for a short walk
- Read—may I suggest you read my books and then re-visit suggestion number one?
- Call a friend—yep, I said *call*, not *text*. Talk to an actual person with your actual voice.
- Express your creativity—paint, sing, play an instrument, dance, write, whatever gets your creative juices flowing!
- Drink some tea—oolong tea actually burns calories and revs up your metabolism.
- Pray—I mean that. If cake is calling to you, maybe Jesus can help. It's worked for me!
- When all else fails, eat a handful of nuts—try it, it really works. Fats stop hunger.

- And perhaps most importantly: learn to be okay with being hungry for a bit.

I know that last one sounds crazy, but one of my biggest victories was simply learning how to cope with my hunger. It actually goes away if you just ignore it for a while, which I didn't know until I was thirty-five years old! Hunger will wane; you should be able to go every three or four hours without a meal. And it's okay to take the time to figure this out for yourself. Feeling hungry doesn't mean you are about to die; it's just a reminder that you will need to eat at some point in the near future.

IMPORTANT TIPS TO BUYING THE BEST FUEL:
- Stay away from anything processed and packaged containing unnatural chemicals—if you can't pronounce the ingredients, don't buy it.
- Farm fresh food is best—try to find a local farmers market you can visit, and don't be afraid to negotiate on the price, especially if you are buying in bulk.
- Customize a meal plan that works best for your family. You'll find you save money by not shopping every day, and sticking to a food plan means you don't have to worry about meal planning until your next shopping cycle.
- Keep an eye on sales of your favorite food items. I know when Zevia goes on sale at my store each month I stock up.
- Try some superfoods! Even your picky eaters might like a few of these, and they are good for you! Some of our favorite superfoods include eggs, walnuts, apples, salmon, canned pumpkin, cauliflower, brown rice, strawberries, black beans, broccoli, sweet potatoes, flaxseed, Greek yogurt, dark chocolate, dried

tart cherries, tea—green and black, natural peanut butter, blackberries, grapes (wine!) and blueberries.

- You don't have to buy *everything* organic, but be aware of the "dirty dozen"— foods that have the highest pesticide residue: peaches, apples, sweet bell peppers, celery, nectarines, strawberries, cherries, pears, imported grapes, spinach, lettuce, and potatoes; you should always buy these organic.

- Always check out the labels of your favorite foods. Is there a better alternative? My youngest son *loves* catsup, so I've switched to one with no added sugar and he likes it just the same—he never even noticed a difference.

- Low-fat, non-fat, and fat-free aren't always a better choice, and sometimes they are actually worse for you, so we usually prefer the full fat and organic options; they taste better, and are better for you.

- I try to use coconut oil whenever I can, as it really is the best and safest option for high heat cooking. The refined version has no coconut taste at all, and you can buy it in spray, liquid, or solid forms to suit your cooking needs. I still use locally made olive oil for lower temp cooking—375 degrees or less to be safe.

- When buying meat, grass-fed or wild is best, and farm fresh is always a wonderful option. Look into farm co-ops near you for great deals on local meat, and check your SAM's Club and Costco for great deals on organic meat.

A quick note about Stevia. When I first started looking into sugar alternatives fifteen or more years ago, there just wasn't much out there. I tried all the alternatives and they all either left me running for the bathroom, bloated, or gassy. I felt pretty awful after several of the protein bars I tried, and don't even get me started on the "diabetic" prepackaged items—they were honestly just gross, and that's putting it nicely.

Now, however, we have stevia, which is 100% natural and comes from the stevia plant. It's one hundred and fifty times sweeter than sugar and it has a negligible affect on blood glucose levels. This sweetener has been a true game changer for me. I've done a lot of research on this, and I believe it to be safe for the whole family—I wouldn't give it to my kids if I thought otherwise. I think this is the best and safest alternative to sugar that we currently have; I've even talked to my doctor, and she agrees. So if your family has a genetic pre-disposition to diabetes, this could be a lifesaver. I use it to modify recipes for baked goods and treats for my family—to rave reviews. Some of my kids even like my baked goods better now than when I made them with regular sugar.

One caveat, however, is that not all stevia sweeteners are created equal. You will even find some "stevia" out there that contains actual sugar in the blend. So beware, that stuff isn't the real, all-natural stevia so don't buy it! I prefer to buy brands that I know and love. We do use a few blends that have xylitol and erythritol in them, but if you use those please be careful with it around your pets, as it can be lethal to dogs if they ingest enough of it. I highly suggest trying the Pyure and Swerve (granular and confectioner type) brands first; my baked goods were greatly improved by the Swerve confectioner's stevia product. But if you don't like those, keep trying until you find one you do like.

A one-to-one to sugar conversion makes things pretty easy to start off with, but your tastes will change the longer you go without sugar, so you might need to keep adjusting the sweetness levels. I'm often scaling back, because things are starting to taste *too* sweet. It's amazing how great these sugar-free treats can be once you find the sweet spot for your family, and if you don't tell your kids it's stevia sweetened, they probably won't even notice! Don't be afraid to take one of your family favorites and give it a go—I think you'll be surprised!

THE NEXT STEP

Once you've finished this book, you're going to start my full eight-week health plan—The Wilder Way. Why eight weeks? Because I believe your body needs time to adjust to the changes you're going to make.

I don't want you focusing on counting calories, points, numbers, or portions. I want you to learn about your body, and discover what *true* health looks and feels like. I'm honestly not sure that the average American even understands what true health means anymore, because we've moved away from natural foods and regular exercise to lead lives that are sedentary and that are fueled, primarily, by processed foods. To compound this issue, we are all confused by what we're being told.

Information has changed so often over the last thirty years that my head has always been spinning: don't eat fat…do eat fat; don't eat carbs…do eat carbs; don't eat eggs…do eat eggs; don't eat red meat, don't ever eat bacon…real meat and bacon is just fine; orange juices causes cancer…orange juice *cures* cancer. Where's the moderate voice in our food culture? And who can be trusted?

Even as I was pouring over recipes, trying to modify them for this book, I ended up throwing many of them out, because either everything was so fancy that none of my kids or my husband would even touch it, or so full of junk that by the time I finished revising the recipe, there was nothing left! Who the hell can get their kids to eat water chestnuts and tofu?

I'm going to show you a new way of eating which at first might sound like nothing you've heard before, something new, something fresh, but I honestly think it's super easy, and makes a whole lot of sense. It might sound a bit overwhelming; I know most of you have a whole family to consider; so winning everyone over can be tough.

I want you to really focus on one meal at a time. That's it. Just focus on that next meal, and make the healthiest choices you can each and every time you sit down to eat. I want this to be fun for you. I want your family to enjoy doing this together. I want them to feel better.

I believe we are on the verge of a food revolution. There's going to be a tipping point where the people suffering from a plethora of food-related diseases will demand change. I think it's coming sooner rather than later, so take the first step with me.

THE BASIC PRINCIPLES OF THE WILDER WAY:

- Eat real foods with minimal ingredients—shoot for five or fewer. If you can't pronounce an ingredient without sounding it out, don't eat it.
- No sugar. None. Nada—Sugar is a killer. No, not even donuts. Say it with me: "SUGAR IS A KILLER!" We'll talk about doing this gradually later on, so for now just keep reading. Don't be scared, you won't even miss it, I promise!
- No processed foods or refined carbohydrates—you only want the real stuff!
- Cycle your food combinations for weight loss—if you want to lose weight, keep your body guessing. More on this later.

- Mindful eating, not mindless eating
- SLEEP—your body needs regular sleep. This is vitally important, so don't skip this one.
- MOVE! Our bodies were made to move. If you want to feel good and look smoking hot, *get moving*! Get up, go outside, and start doing your thing, whatever it may be. More on this later, as well.
- As always, be sure to stay hydrated!

So why isn't my program complicated? Aren't diets supposed to be complicated? Don't we need to suffer? Why aren't there little boxes to measure your serving sizes? Why don't you have to count calories?

Why?

Well, I think that's all bullshit. Sorry if that's a little blunt, but I've been counting calories my whole life. I've counted points and calories, I've used boxes and pre-packaged servings, and all of this got me exactly nowhere. It didn't accomplish one thing. So, if none of that worked, why are those methods still out there? Why are we still gaining weight? Why is our health crisis getting worse each day? Why are there more and more obese Americans every year?

We need to stop focusing on another weight loss program or exercise gimmick. Instead, we need to focus on something totally different: our food choices. It's really that simple. All it really takes is reading labels, and a little knowledge. My plan is for busy women—and men too!—who just want to be able to spend their precious time with their kids, and not measuring, boxing, or counting bullshit points systems or calories.

My plan is taking us back to the basics. Nourishing food, physical movement, and health. That's it! Sit back and relax. If a mom of six with a farm and a publishing business can do this, you can too!

Pro tip: I never leave my house without filling my purse with snacks; now I never get sidetracked by the pastry window at Starbucks. I don't leave home without some nuts, a Quest bar, or some dark chocolate...or all three!

Chapter 12

THE WINE DIET: CHOCOLATE, WINE, AND SEX...
ALL IMPORTANT FOOD GROUPS

"All you need is love. But a little chocolate now and then doesn't hurt."
— Charles M. Schulz

THIS IS A SPECIAL LITTLE CHAPTER FOR ALL THE COUPLES OUT there. If you aren't married, or in a committed relationship, move on to the next chapter. Move on, move on, there's nothing to see here.

If you are married or committed, then grab a glass of your favorite wine and let's chat for a moment.

My husband and I *love* what we do. We have a passion for reading, writing, marriage and sex. Luckily for us, all those things go together and, from chatting with many of our readers, it does for them too! We hope to share more of our marriage wisdom in its own full book one day, but for now I just wanted to add a special chapter on how food, marriage, how we feel about ourselves and life in general all seem to interconnect for so many women. After I wrote *Big Girls Do It Better*, I was literally overwhelmed with emails from women who told me they were having sex with their husbands regularly after a long period of going without it. That was so exciting to me!

There are many reasons you might experience a sexual drought in your marriage. Maybe you had a new baby, or one of you is struggling with illness. Maybe one or both of you are under a lot of stress from work. Maybe finances have you in knots. Maybe you just feel like shit about yourself, and simply don't have the desire.

The really worrisome thing about many of the emails I received is how women just felt too bad about themselves and their bodies to enjoy sex with their husbands—they were ashamed of their bodies. Ladies, this is unacceptable! If there's one thing that'll put a marriage at risk for divorce, it's that.

I'm sure if you asked your husband right now, he would be up for sex with you no matter what state you are in. Heck, I once went to the bathroom post-sex to find mascara smeared all over my face and I looked like a raccoon. My husband didn't seem to mind at all—I'm not even sure he noticed! My body is covered in scars from surgery, I've lost and gained a few hundred pounds, and my breasts have fed five babies. I'm sure you get the picture.

My point is you need to get your sexy back!

Your husband *needs* sex with you, and you *need* sex with him! Sex is incredibly important to your overall health, on top of just being fun, so grab a glass of red wine (lots of wonderful antioxidants!), some dark chocolate (superfood!), and get into the bedroom for some "exercise" with your husband. I even read recently that some studies have been done showing wine can actually help with weight loss—yippie!

I can honestly say I've never laughed as much or come as hard as after a nightcap of good wine and a few bites of dark chocolate shared with Mr. Wilder. Sometimes we get really crazy and challenge each other to planking or push up contests and then jump into bed.

The best part about this is that you are also going to burn some calories having sex—up to two hundred calories when you have a *really* good time! Now, if I was worried about how I looked, or if I didn't feel sexy, or how I looked or felt inside, I would miss out on all that marital fun.

If that's you, then you need to listen up.

Mama, you *deserve* that love and attention from your man. My goal is to get you feeling better about yourself, so you'll want it, and know deep down that your man thinks you're sexy. Little steps will make all the difference in how you feel, so start eating better, get moving, and take good care of yourself. All of these things are connected.

When you feel better inside, you'll want to show that on the outside. Don't miss out on life, don't let it pass you by because you think you can't do this—you can! Sex is a part of the whole program. Regardless of what size you are today, or how you're feeling about your body just remember, tomorrow is a new day. Being relaxed and having fun with your husband will only make this journey so much better for *both* of you.

Personally, I'm not in favor of depriving myself in any way. There are days where I'm just pushing through to get to the wine and chocolate part of the night. With six kids and a hundred farm animals all running amok, those treats are sometimes what helps me keep hold on my sanity; this is something that took me a long time to figure out. What's on the outside reflects what's inside, and what's inside you is reflected outside, so fake it till you make it, if that's what it takes. On the days when I'm feeling down, or I just feel like crap, I put on some lipstick and sexy panties. I know it sounds crazy and almost *too* simple, but those two things can help you get into a slightly different frame of mind. Maybe paint your toenails or wear your favorite color, or put that lipstick and those panties on, take a photo and send it to your hubby. Whatever it takes! Just don't let yourself think you aren't a sexual being—*you are*. Marriages need sex. Daddy needs sex. Mama needs sex… and maybe some wine and chocolate too. Don't worry: you don't even have to report back to me on this one. Just do your thing, and maybe name the baby Jasinda.

I'm kidding…mostly. If Lily's chocolates wanted to change the name of their sea salt chocolate to the Jasinda Bar, I would totally understand. Eat one and you'll see what I mean. They're that good!

MY FAVORITE WAYS TO INDULGE AND FEEL SEXY:

- A nice hot bubble bath—add a LUSH bath bomb for extra luxuriousness. Those things are magic!
- A nice box of Dr. John's chocolates. These things are sugar-free and you'd never know it. Give them a try and thank me later: www.drjohns.com
- LELO brand personal pleasure products. No need to thank me if you don't already know about these. Wow. Just…*wow*.
- Oil candles. We just got some of these as a gift and the wax actually dissolves into a massage oil. Very sexy and really sets a sultry mood.
- Spanx. Yep, I know. I might get some backlash for this, but I actually love my Spanx. I've been known to wear them to bed for sexy time. They help me feel good and tuck in my mommy belly—I think they put the hole in the crotch for multiple reasons. There's no shame in putting those on for a night out if you want to get everything pushed up and held in so you feel good for yourself and look good for your man.
- Music or audiobooks! Sex is all about the senses, so put on

your favorite sexy tunes, or make your husband a playlist and send it to him. Maybe you like to listen to your favorite hot book before bed. Hey, the couple that listens together gets busy together!

- Speaking of which…read any of our Jack and/or Jasinda Wilder books to get in the mood. We love it when you invite us into your bedroom…metaphorically speaking.

Chapter 13

BIG GIRL PSYCHOLOGY 101

BEFORE WE GO ANY FURTHER, I THINK IT'S IMPORTANT WE TOUCH on some "Big Girl" thinking. I've been morbidly obese for nearly twenty-five years. That's a very long time to deal with everything that goes along with being a big girl. And let's just put it all out in the open: there's a lot that comes with being overweight. I believe it's one of the last things that people will still publicly ridicule and mock.

I follow a very successful plus size model that I've seen called every single nasty name in the book, *publicly*, on her professional social media pages. It's honestly disgusting. Why do people think this is okay? It's not! We are more than our bodies. We are also souls, sometimes delicate and always beautiful, souls. You never know what someone has gone through, or is going through, because of their weight.

Shame on our society for taking their own pain, anger and frustration out on people with weight issues. We've heard all the jokes and names and none of it was ever funny, so just stop already.

I believe this shaming has put women—especially women in the public eye—into one of two categories: one group are the women who say, "Eff you, I'm going to look however I want to look. I'm big and I'm proud of it!" Category two is the group that says, "Let's not talk about the elephant in the room that is my weight."

As a woman, it's very difficult not to let yourself be defined in some way by your body, regardless of your size, but it's exponentially harder for women who are curvy or plus-sized. Some of the questions I've been asked about my books tip toe around the idea that I wrote a "BBW" series. Honestly, I hate categorizing my books and I'm not a huge fan of the BBW title. When I wrote the *Big Girls* series, I was honestly just writing my own story. It didn't even really occur to me that Anna was a "plus sized heroine" until people pointed it out to me. I just wanted to tell that particular story about that particular girl at that moment in time. Who knows what she looks like now or what she's doing now? Hopefully, she's happy and feeling good.

I'm not sure which side of the coin most of my readers are on, so my reason for writing this book is to share where I've been, what I'm going through, and where I hope to end up. At this point in my life, my happiness has very little to do with looks. I figure I'm a bit past my prime and too happily married to worry about it. My focus at this point in my life is my health.

As a society, I would love to see us make peace with our bodies and make peace with each other.

I know that some of my readers have been pretty vocal to me about their success with gastric bypass and band surgeries, so I'm going to address that as well. I found lots of staggering statistics while I was researching this book. The truth is, less than 20% of people who undergo those procedures keep the weight off for more than a few years. Many of them have additional health problems arising from the surgery, and more than 10% require additional operations after the first surgery. A recent study by the National Institutes of Health showed almost 40% end up having serious complications or nutritional deficiencies.

I know there are exceptions to every rule but in my mind, surgical procedures are just putting a Band-Aid on a gaping wound. Simply cutting people open and removing part of their intestines can't solve our nation's obesity problem. Why aren't we more successful with those procedures? Well, I believe that the body, mind and soul are all connected, and those surgeries only address a single aspect of the weight problem, and not even permanently or safely for that matter. Surgical procedures that modify our bodies won't change our brains, our habits, the way we think about ourselves, or what we eat.

When I volunteered at a well-known bariatric hospital after my surgery, I saw a lot of horrible things, like people trading food addictions for addictions to alcohol, drugs, and sex, and I saw people coming in for their second or *third* bypass or banding. People who are so desperate for health end up more frustrated, without hope, and in worse shape than they were before their surgeries.

I believe eating right and dealing with our emotions and connections to food is critical for success. You *must* break the chains food has over your body and mind. Success comes through strength. If you've had bypass surgery and gained the weight back, it's okay, that doesn't define you! If you plan to undergo that surgery, I wish you the best of luck with it but, *please,* do the research and understand it's just a tool and, in my opinion, an unsafe one. There is a better, safer, long-term solution. Not all doctors will tell you that, either—mine didn't. Bariatric surgery is an extremely lucrative business, one which doctors and hospitals make enormous profits from.

Love your body the best you can. Give it a chance to get healthy without putting it at even greater risk. Please keep reading this book. I would love to show you a safer way. Let's heal from the inside out. If you've already had a surgical intervention and still need help to feel good and healthy, please join me.

We can do this!

In the next chapter of this book I'm going to focus on physical strength, wellness, and health. I want to be very clear though, and say that none of the things I have accomplished changes the fact that I will always be a Big Girl who puts on her big girl panties every single day. I'm a touch under six feet tall and I have a size twelve and a half shoe. My frame just isn't tiny, and that's how God made me. It's part of who I am—heck, it is *who* I am.

But, regardless of my weight, I'm a woman, and one with serious health issues, some which stem from my own poor choices, but still more from being misinformed. The last year was an epiphany for me; I've learned so much, not just about myself, but also about the human body. I want you to know that no matter what your weight may be; you can *always* be healthier by making positive food choices, engaging in physical movement and getting enough rest. We are all works in progress. Yes, I've lost a significant amount of weight making these changes, but even more importantly, I've found my strength and my health. I've discovered pride in my body.

I recently ran five miles without stopping... *five* miles! Can you believe that? I honestly couldn't believe it even while I was actually doing it. It's *nuts*! I've always had asthma and bad knees, even as a child. How the hell could I run that far —albeit slowly—without stopping?

What I realized was that I've been lying to myself my whole life. I just assumed I couldn't do it. Fat kids can't run, and fat adults certainly can't, so how could I do it now? Thirty-six years old, mother of six children, countless health issues; there's just no way, right? Well, what if all those lies are silenced once I clean the toxins out my body? What if my body starts working in concert with my mind, and I start to believe I *can* do it? What then?

That's where this is headed.

So, get on your running shoes and take my hand. This isn't just *my* moment, it's also *yours*. There's a reason I'm writing this book right now: it's for *YOU*. Today is the day, *NOW* is the time. You are going to get moving with me. We've been fed a bunch of bullshit and told a lifetime of lies, and now it's time to fight back. We've been abused, made fun of, yelled at, and looked down upon. Not anymore, my friend. This is when our tiger comes out and we stop letting this abuse go any further.

I don't care if your whole closet is full of BBW pride T-shirts and you're standing strong for the positive body image cause—that's wonderful, but don't let your health suffer for it. Let's continue to fight for *all* women, but for ourselves first.

Good health and change starts with *you*. You have more power than you think! Mama, you've got the power to change the course of the rest of your life.

If you are hearing lies in your head, stop now and say this out loud with me—yes, actually say it out loud. If your family is home and you are embarrassed just go into your bathroom.

Stand in front of the mirror and say this out loud:

"God meant for my body to be healthy and strong.

I am worth the time it will take to make myself stronger and healthier.

It won't be easy, but it will be worth it.

Yes, it's okay to do this for those who love me, but this is for me.

I was beautiful then, I am beautiful now, and I will be beautiful tomorrow.

I can do this.

I can do this despite feeling like I can't, or that I've been told I can't.

My body is beautiful at any size.

My body is going to be unstoppable when I'm healthier and stronger, so watch out!

Nothing will define me.

Nothing will stop me.

I can do this!"

PART 3

Running Wild!

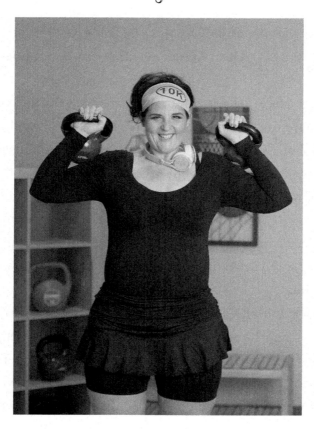

Chapter 14

THE CHALLENGE

"Run when you can, walk if you have to, crawl if you must; just never give up." — Dean Karnazes, ultramarathon runner

I'M ABOUT TO CHALLENGE YOU. ACTUALLY, I'M GOING TO FULL-ON *double* dare you to run with me, and by run I mean walk, wog, jog, wobble, hobble, whatever it takes you to get to the finish line. I'm not kidding; I'm not even sort of joking about this. I want you to get on Google *right now* and find a 5k race in your area. Maybe there's one coming up in a few weeks, maybe there's one happening in a few months. Either way, I know you're laughing and thinking, "There is *no* freaking way I'm going to do this! Jasinda Wilder has obviously lost her mind."

Truth be told, I lost it long, long ago, but I'm not joking about this. This is a real, honest to goodness, throw-down challenge. I want you to do this. Not because I told you to, but because there is a tiny little speck of *"just maybe I can"* hiding inside you somewhere.

Don't worry about being ready, because you never will be. You just have to do it, ready or not.

So go ahead and sign yourself up for your very first 5k.

Yes, right now.

I'll wait.

Jasinda Wilder

Still waiting.

This is not a joke; and, yes, your friend can come too.

Sure, sign up your whole family without asking them, like I did.
They'll love you for it…I promise.

What are you waiting for? You can do this. Come on!

Whew, I'm so glad you did that! I was worried we would lose time on this.

Now I can officially say you're in training with me. This is the blind leading the blind, the wogger leading the woggie—"wog" is what I call my "walk-jog." It's a low impact run I do to protect my knees. I'll explain more about that later, the important part is that now you're ready for some serious training.

The next few chapters are basically going to be an idiot's guide to getting moving. Registering for a 5k is half the work, so consider yourself half done. Now, let's get to the really fun stuff!

I know, I know, right now it might actually feel like suicide to attempt this. Me? Run five kilometers? That's like…three miles! Three point one, to be exact, but I know you can do this, and I know when you reach the finish line you'll go home and sign up for the next chance to reach the finish line. You may never have thought of yourself as a runner, but guess what? You are, now! Your body was built to move. It was built to run, jump, dance, and walk. It's part of the design. You are, in fact, a born runner.

When my family started feeling better, we decided we wanted to create some memories doing physical things together. We had seen on Facebook that a local running club was sponsoring several 5k runs to benefit charities throughout the upcoming fall and winter holidays. One of the wonderful things about our local community is that most of the runs sponsor a local charity, so not only are you helping yourself get stronger and healthier, but you're also helping a local charity, so it's a win/win!

I know a lot of people think these events are only for the uber-athletic, but let me tell you; those types blaze to the end as soon as the gun goes off. Like, they're done and home having a snack by the time I reach the finish line. The people I roll with are moms with strollers, senior citizens, and fat dogs. In fact, during one race a very fat dog with a limp jogged right past me—honest-to-God truth! My point is, you don't have to be the fastest. You don't even have to be in the top fifty percent. Everyone gets a shirt or a hat, and everyone can have whatever time he or she needs to finish. I'm sure someone out there is thinking they'll be dead last. So what? At least you did it! You're doing more than someone who's at home in front of the TV. What did they gain that morning? Nothing! But you…you're a finisher! You are one badass mother runner! You did your first 5k!

Your first one is going to be special and maybe a bit crazy, because you don't know what to expect. The wonderful thing is that there will be other first-timers there, too. You won't be the only one and you certainly don't need to be embarrassed. You'll be able to tell the real athletes from the…not-athletes, trust me on this one. All sorts of different people will be there, and there'll always be someone there to cheer you on.

I'll never forget our Jingle Run, a 5k we did around Christmastime. I was pushing our baby in a stroller while dragging my four-year-old who was in desperate need of a nap. We were nearing the end of the race—thank God!—when a person on the side of the road watching the race yelled, "Wow, she's jammin'!" They were talking about me! I was jammin'! He may have been talking about the fact that I was blasting "Turn Down For What" on my phone's speakers as loud as it would go, but I prefer to think he was talking about my amazing 16 minutes per mile pace.

Please don't worry about your time for your first race, or doing too much training—I don't want you to worry about that at all, in fact. Just commit to doing it, even if you have to walk the whole thing. My older daughter sometimes walks while I wog and she finishes before I do! Do this at your pace and no one else's. The only person you're competing against is yourself. There's no shame in getting there when you get there, whether it's in thirty minutes or two hours! If you can do short bursts of speed to pick up the pace, hey, that's great. I just want you to get out there and *do it*. Don't get overwhelmed and don't go overboard.

Don't get ahead of yourself. This is important to understand. Don't make this yet another New Year's resolution to change your life. I want you to stick with this for more than a day or a week or a month, or even a year; this is your new forever. We're going to take this one step at a time. Maybe you want to work on your food plan first and get things going there. My mom has been doing that for months without really increasing her exercise at all, and she's had amazing results. I didn't start moving until I felt better and knew it was time to move.

So what does that look like for you? This isn't one size fits all. Maybe you need to move first and then adjust your food plan. In my experience, though, cutting out the worst enemies to your health is a great place to start, and then gradually make other changes.

Physical exercise and strength training *is* important; I do want to make that very clear. I read several diet books that basically said exercise was optional and not that important. I don't buy that for a second.

Why?

Because of what I've seen and experienced with my own body.

I really believe nutrition and physical fitness go hand and hand with feeling great and looking great. Could we probably excel in one without the other? Yeah, sure. I just heard about a trainer with an amazing body and huge social media following who says she eats almost only fast food. Hmmmm…that doesn't make much sense to me. Why trash the inside of your body and then work so hard on the outside? Let's find a balance and love both the inside *and* the outside. They both deserve your attention, right? I want you healthy—body, mind and soul!

So how do we really get started on a lifestyle of physical fitness? I'm not talking about becoming a gym rat or running in circles all weekend, I'm talking about adjusting your life in increments to make your exercise and physical wellness a priority as well as something fun. How does that look for you? For me it means a few things. I spend half of my day on my feet—at least 8,000 to 10,000 steps every day however I can get them in, and I do some sort of fun exercise for thirty minutes, four to five days a week.

This can take the form of a bunch of different things—a fast paced walk or run with my kids, a YouTube video with some cardio dance moves to a popular song, working a simple Kettlebell circuit, hell, even just walking up and down my stairs a few times. I do whatever I can, each and every day, to get my body moving.

If you have a home office or have any influence at work, I highly suggest either a standing desk or a walking desk. I have a walking treadmill desk I use every single day. If you see me on social media, it's almost always when I'm on my treadmill desk, because it's a great way to kill two birds with one stone. I get my steps in, keep my back in good shape, answer emails, and even edit my books while at my treadmill desk. Those steps each day really hold me accountable to staying on track with my work while benefitting my health.

A quick aside to all of my author friends who might be reading this—get a walking desk, PLEASE. A sedentary life spent sitting down all day every day is not good for your body. I do a fast walk or wog while I'm doing my social media and emails, and then a nice slow stroll while I am writing. You'll be surprised how quickly that will get you off

social media, and how many miles you'll be walking in a day. Hell, I
challenge you to sprint with me! Message me and we can word-sprint
while physically challenging each other to see who can walk the farthest
or fastest. All that hard work won't be worth much if you're sick, so
please take care of yourself. Please move, and eat well. Our profession
worries me, because we're all too isolated and stationary. Get moving!
Let's be leaders in our industry. Let's get ourselves in fighting shape! We
need you to be healthy so we can keep reading your books.

Sorry, but that needed to be said.

Now, I know a walking desk is specific to my life and job, but I
bet you can find ways to make double tasking work for you. The other day I came across a group of mommy fitness bloggers who incorporate their kids' play time with their workouts. They hold their kids
while doing squats, and/or use them as extra weights for pushups. I
don't know if that would work with my crazy kids, but I might just
give it a try when I'm in a pinch for some extra free weight—gotta
put those kids to use somehow! My point is, there *has* to be some extra things you can do to stay active. You'll be surprised at how much
extra energy it gives you, and how much better you'll sleep at night.
Also, don't underestimate those bathroom break squats.

I signed up for my first 5k not long after my oldest daughter
was born. My friend, who's super athletic and has been running her
whole life, told me to do a training program first, but of course I
didn't listen. Why would I? I never do what anyone tells me...just
ask Jack! I think I'd run a total of two times for five minutes at most
before driving to downtown Detroit for the 5k run I'd promised my
friend I would do with her.

I wasn't in any kind of shape to do it, but I was sure as hell going
to pretend. As soon as the race started I *blazed* to the very start of the

pack. It may have been more of a hobble, but it felt like I was blazing. I got about a mile into the race when I started to realize this might actually be the day I died.

I tried to slow down, but when you're in the middle of a pack of actual runners, people who know what they're doing, people who can actually run faster than a stroll, it's kind of hard to stop, or even slow down. You'll get trampled like the running of the bulls in Pamplona. So, of course, I did what any self-respecting person who's trying not to die during a race would do: I pretended I had a horrible cramp. Actually, I didn't have to pretend… I did have multiple cramps…shit, my whole body was one giant cramp, and I couldn't breathe. It was a bitterly cold November day in Detroit, so my lungs hadn't adjusted, and I was literally hyperventilating.

What the blue fuck had I been thinking? I'm pretty sure I actually saw Jesus for a minute; I was *that* close to death. So I collapsed to the ground and just stayed there for a couple of minutes and tried to catch my breath. After a while I was finally able to get some oxygen into my lungs, at which point all the normal, non-running people were starting to appear at the rear of the pack. These were *my* people, I realized. The great thing was that there were people doing a brisk walk and others who were just strolling—*this* I could handle. I ended up finishing that race with a grand time of 58 minutes.

Here's the deal, though. Someone out there may have been laughing at me, but I was pretty proud of that finishing time. I had actually finished! I conquered those three point one miles, and I did it in the freaking cold and snow no less! And I hadn't even trained! Just imagine what I could have done had I actually taken some time for preparation.

Now, you might think that experience would have inspired me to continue on doing more 5ks. Well…it didn't. I was happy just to still be alive. I thought, "Wow, God kept me here on the Earth, so I probably shouldn't attempt anything that dumb ever again."

It wouldn't be until years later that I even *thought* about doing another one. Why? Because it's easier not to—and that's the honest to goodness truth. It's much easier to stay home in a warm bed and just relax on a Saturday morning, whereas it takes real effort to wake up early, get suited up, and actually run a race.

Let's go back to what I was saying earlier about what you're eating. A good portion of my life was spent struggling against a food haze. Even when I was trying to eat right, things I didn't even know were bad for me were causing so many problems. I was in a constant food coma, and didn't even realize it. Most people are in that same place right now, I think. Just floating along in an impenetrable food coma caused by a lifetime of poor nutrition, simply because they don't know any better.

Imagine spending years eating a whole-wheat bagel with low fat cream cheese, fruit, and fruit-on-the-bottom yogurt, only to find out those foods are actually doing *serious* damage to your body. That was my problem, that's your problem…that's our whole nation's problem. Once I changed the way I ate and the order in which I ate food—BAM! I had *unbelievable* energy. I was doing things that "those people" did, those athletic go-getter lunatics I've always hated! Running five or six miles, lifting kettlebells, jumping rope, doing interval sprints... and best of all, I didn't feel as if I was about to die afterwards.

We've all heard the stereotype that fat people are lazy. Man, I've always hated that crap. Because you know what? I wasn't *lazy*, I was being *poisoned*. I know that might sound shocking or melodramatic, but it's true. Take away all that sugar, all that processed, mutated, and refined carbohydrate crap and *WHAM!* You're gonna to feel like a new person!

This is vitally important, supremely important. You *have* to kick that poisonous bullshit to the curb before you're going to see real success with your walking, moving, and running.

I have energy to do things I never thought was possible, and I believe you do, too!

So, how do we get started? Well, you could download one of those running apps, or you could hire a personal trainer, or any number of other possibilities, but what I think you should do just *start moving.* That's it. Just move. Five minutes a day, if that's all you can handle at first. Whatever, however long. It doesn't matter. Just *move.*

Ideally, you should be moving for thirty consecutive minutes, three to four times a week. I started with walking. Please, don't go crazy and hurt yourself! Remember, your body is still healing and we don't want to derail that, so start with something you like, something basic and fun, and over time your body will start telling you when it's ready for more.

I spent weeks just strolling slowly while answering emails at my walking treadmill desk. Sometimes I would increase the pace for a while and then slow it back down. I would make it a game to see how much walking I could do in thirty minutes. How far could I go, how fast could I go? Then I started gradually increasing the pace until I reached the max the treadmill would allow, but this happened about two months after starting my new nutritional program, not in the first week, or even in the first month. I just knew my body felt stronger and I felt ready to push a bit more, so I started wogging.

Wogging is just a low impact walk, but at a slightly faster pace. Sort of a combination between walking and jogging. I try to hit the ground with the middle of my foot and not raise my legs very high so I can protect my knees, which aren't in the best shape.

Listen to your body. Set goals and select races you would love to run. You'd be amazed what a powerful motivation it is to know you've committed to a race. I really believe that *everyone* can finish a 5k. For example, this past New Year's Day, my entire extended family ran one together. My sixty-year-old in-laws both beat me to the finish line! And you know what? I was as proud as I could be! Running that race with their grandparents is a great memory my kids will have forever.

Now, get out there and move!

FROM COUCH TO 5K IN 20 DAYS:
Day 1—locate several pairs of yoga pants
Day 2—put on your best pair of yoga pants
Day 3—locate your running shoes
Day 4—realize you don't own running shoes
Day 5—go to a good retailer or get on Amazon and buy some good running shoes; don't skimp on the shoes, because taking care of your feet is key to consistent running.
Day 6—put on yoga pants, running bra, a shirt, new running shoes, and take a sexy selfie. Now take a nap, because that shit was exhausting.
Day 7—it's raining and you don't want your hair to get wet. Not running.
Day 8—get suited up and run one block. Almost die. Go home.
Day 9—get suited up and run two blocks. You're going to need headphones to do this again.
Day 10—get on Amazon and one-click some Beats head-phones—so worth the price!
Day 11—block one actually didn't seem all that bad! I'm killing it!

Day 12—block three killed me. I'm dead. Walk home and take a nap.

Day 13—run four blocks without stopping! YES!

Day 14—run six blocks without stopping!

Day 15—take a day off. Running is hard.

Day 16—take another day off because it's hard to get upright after all that stupid running.

Day 17—run eight blocks and pass the neighbor's fat dog that's out for a walk.

Day 18—run nine blocks at a speed *almost* faster than walking. Almost, but not quite.

Day 19—run ten blocks with only two stops to stave off imminent death.

Day 20—run the full ten blocks without stopping even once. If you can do that, you'll totally kill a 5K. You're always allowed to walk if you need to, and there are usually snacks at the end. You've got this!

That was a joke, but not really—any effort put into being healthy is worthwhile. Each day you try to do something, *anything*, in an attempt to be healthier is a step in the right direction. No one expects you to become an ultra-marathoner, or try out for the Olympics. I just want you to *make the effort*. Your body was made to move. You're strong and you're ready, *right now*. There's nothing more important than your health, so even if it's just a walk from the far end of the parking lot into the store, take it. Think of each step as a step in the right direction. Take that extra time and do something good for yourself. You'll never know what you're capable of until you try, and my guess is if we give you one 5k, you're going to want at least four more to go with it. Once we have the ball rolling, you're going to be unstoppable. So, lace up those cute running shoes and let's get moving.

You've got some races to run!

Chapter 15

YES, RUNNING SUCKS BUT IT'S ALSO SORT OF AWESOME

I HATE RUNNING. HONESTLY, I DO. I HATE HAVING TO PUT ON ALL these stupid special clothes and shoes. I mean, running requires wearing pants! Who wants to wear pants? There's no part of me that really ever feels *excited* about going out to run. The entire time I'm getting ready I'm thinking, "Why the hell am I doing this to myself?" Well, maybe there *is* a tiny part of me that gets excited when I run with my husband; it is fun to watch his cute little butt running up the hill in front of me. But, other than that, it never seems like a great idea.

When I'm actually running, or "wogging", I hate it even more. I'm sweaty, I'm out of breath, cars full of people who might know me are passing by left and right, and body parts I didn't even know I had are chafing.

Even though our ancestors have been running for ages, running for exercise still seems about as logical as juggling porcupines na-ked…while walking a tightrope. Maybe not *that* bad, but still pretty awkward.

The key to learning how to do anything is to take it slow and build up your awesomeness in stages. The first time you run, literally just try to walk a block to get warmed up to the idea, and then wog until you can't wog anymore. For me, that stage went on for weeks. My nanny would send me texts at least once a day asking if I was okay because apparently she thought I was dying, based on the noises I was making. Even if you sound like a donkey in labor, the chances of you actually dying are actually pretty slim, so just trust me when I say that if *I* can do it, you can too!

You'll be cursing me for the first few weeks, I'm sure, but I'm also willing to wager you'll start feeling better and stronger, and that your endurance will increase with time and effort. It's amazing how quickly we can stop feeling like crap and start feeling like Wonder Woman once we put our mind to it.

If you're only able to walk, just try to increase your walking pace a little. Maybe you start with trying to do a twenty-minute mile and in the first few weeks make it your goal to get that down to seventeen or eighteen minutes. That's great! When you walk, jog, or run, the only person you are competing with is yourself.

When I first started running, I made notes on my iPhone to keep track of my progress; each day I would note the day, time, and how far and how fast I walked or wogged. And in just in a few weeks I could see a *huge* improvement. I also started to notice the shape of my body changing, and I knew I was getting stronger. I could pick up my son more easily, and I wasn't out of breath walking up a flight or two of stairs. I was even sleeping better!

The increase in energy was remarkable right off the bat. Being able to exercise was a direct, immediate result of hauling my ass out of the sugar haze. I was a better wife, mother, and writer because my mind and body just simply *felt better.*

This is really important; because I think as women we can easily get sucked into a pretty vicious cycle. If we don't feel good, we take even worse care of ourselves, which leads us down a rabbit hole of eating more, and eating nasty, unhealthy crap, because what's the point, right? If we're gonna feel like shit and look like shit, why bother? Sometimes we feel like we won't ever get back to where we once were. We can't seem to break the cycle, and that donut or that ice cream bar makes us feel a tiny bit better for a few minutes. But then, almost immediately, it makes us feel worse physically and we get down on ourselves mentally for being weak. Then we're right back into the cycle again.

Our American life often makes it hard to recover from these things. We watch *The Biggest Loser* or *Extreme Weight Loss*, which leads us to think the only way we can break out of the cycle is to throw our whole life at it, to sign up for the gym and lift weights and shake ropes and flip tires and eat nothing but celery and tofu and water chestnuts.

Well, I don't know about you, but the thought of that seems pretty freaking exhausting to me. I get tired and hungry and irritable just *watching* those programs. What I think is missing in so many of these approaches is the idea of taking things slow and steady. Taking things one day at a time, one meal at a time. Rome wasn't built in one day. Your body didn't get this way in one day, and it certainly won't get healthy again in one day…or even in one week, or one month!

The good news is that even if you lose just *half* a pound each week, that's twenty-five pounds lost in a year. Lose a whole pound a week and you've just kissed fifty pounds goodbye in a year. With that weight loss will come increased strength, wellness, mental clarity and increased energy. You're going to *feel* like getting up and getting moving, and you will feel as if you've actually, finally, got a handle on things.

I've learned that most good things in life are worth waiting for, worth working for, and that anything worth having usually doesn't come overnight, so start small. List your goals and cross them off one by one, day by day.

You're *worth* it. You're worth the time it will take to make this happen. Your health is the most important thing in your life, so take the time and make the effort, every single day.

I know moms out there are asking, "What about my family? What about my kids?" And my response is, how can you take care of those precious babies if you aren't feeling well all the time? You can't! So take some time out for yourself, get your health in order, get yourself feeling great and looking great.

As far as running goes, I've got lots of goals. I want to finish my first 10k with my three oldest kids and my husband, running my fastest time ever. The thought of running six point two miles scares the literal poop out of me but, damn it, I'm determined to try! Second, I want to continue to get better at this. I want to be a positive example for my kids. I want to show them that even Mom can get into "beast mode" at the end of a race, and sprint that last tenth of a mile. I want them to see that health is a priority for me and, by extension, a priority for them.

If you're a mom and you're reading this, I encourage you to get your kids out there with you. These are family memories they'll have for their whole lives. You'll laugh, wog, and cry together. Even my little kids talk about how awesome our "turkey race" was last Thanksgiving. (I haven't heard a single mention of the yummy sugar-free pie I made that day, but the race itself is brought up in family conversation all the time). These are things they won't forget, and you're leaving them a legacy of health, too. A healthy mom is more likely to have healthy kids who, in turn, become healthy adults. Plus, it's just plain fun to run together.

Here's something that I don't hear people talk much about either: when you finish a run—I don't care if it's a community 5k or just a run around your neighborhood—you're going to feel *good*. And not just sorta good, a million bucks good! The more you do it, the better it feels. It's almost like good wine, or sex. Regular physical activity will give you a stronger mind and an increased sense of wellbeing.

My kids keep telling me how much better they feel, how much more soundly they sleep. Even on days when they kick and scream about it, as soon as we get out there they talk about how much they love it when we run. If you don't have kids, take your husband, or your boyfriend, a friend, your dog, your mom, or heck, even drag a second cousin along with you—having a pal when you run always makes it more enjoyable.

When my family runs, we break off into groups, and those who reach the finish line first cheer on the stragglers. The weekends when we have a run are always so much fun. My kids fight less, they are more focused and they are kinder to each other.

Go ahead and test me on this. You can thank me later. Maybe one day we can all race together. Wouldn't that be fun?

Another benefit from this increase in health and stamina is in the area of marital relations. I'm sure I don't have to spell it all out, but once you become more physically fit that part of your marriage will be…healthier, let's say. So let hubby in on that little secret when he starts complaining that you signed the whole family up for a run. There are benefits for all! Trust me!

Below are few other benefits of running and overall physical fitness:

- You'll sleep better.
- You'll be happier. You'll feel amazing, even after a short run.

Try just doing twenty minutes and see if you don't feel better, even if you've had a rough day. I would bet money you'll want to do it again tomorrow. There's science behind this—it's been proven that running releases dopamine.

- Your body will be leaner. It may take some time, but you'll see your body start to change. It will make you stronger and you'll add muscle one step at a time. And, you can burn eight hundred and fifty calories per hour!

- Increased strength and endurance. If you have bad knees, walking and wogging will make them stronger. I know that many of us bigger people worry about our knees, so trust me when I say that even if your knees make lots of strange noises, like mine do, it will get better as you run more—I can't believe how well mine have held up.

- Reduced risk of cancer. There's scientific proof of this, too. Don't believe me? Google it! Why wouldn't you want to get moving if it could aid you in the fight against cancer?

- You'll live longer. Again, science!

- Relief from anxiety and depression. For some it's almost like meditation, and it's certainly better than medication. I know this sounds weird, but it does put you in a chill mind space.

- Stronger lungs and heart. Yes, I was the fat kid with asthma, but running has actually helped my lung strength and increased my stamina.

- Increased confidence and body image. You'll feel more badass with every mile you put under your feet. There's no better feeling than crossing a finish line, or meeting a goal you've set for yourself.

Chapter 16

SO YOU STILL THINK YOU CAN'T RUN?

"What if I fall? Oh but my darling, what if you fly?" — Erin Hanson

I CAN ALREADY HEAR YOU INSISTING YOU CAN'T DO IT. IN FACT, I hear it when I'm running, too. If you put a hundred women in a line-up and asked them to step forward if they think their body is banging, I'd be surprised if more than a handful take that step forward. I think our society places value on things most women can never live up to. We're constantly being told we have to be shredded, that we should be tiny in some places and unnaturally large in others. We see entertainers shot full of Botox and silicone and think we're less beautiful and badass than them because we sag and have wrinkles and cellulite, and they don't. How do we turn this around? How can we empower our daughters and sons to look elsewhere for standards of true beauty? How can we display better values?

Ladies, this revolution starts at home. It starts with you. It starts with me. It starts with your mom, your aunt, your daughter, your best friend and your neighbor. It starts here and now.

I just want to digress for a moment. My family watches very little TV. We have one television in our home, and it's in a family area where we all have to agree on one program. It's also way upstairs, a bit out of the way, so we have to actually get up and move if we want to watch something. This was a conscious choice for us. Why? Because we want to see what our kids are watching. Does that mean we're constantly helicoptering over every single thing they are exposed to? No. But it does put us within earshot if they see something depicting women, relationships, or life in a way we don't agree with and then we can start a conversation about it.

This isn't the perfect solution, but it does keep conversations with our kids open and honest about things like how people look and how they are perceived, what people think, what they say, and why. Talking with your kids is important. I don't really try to hide things from them—I want them to form their own opinions and not be negatively influenced by society's views, especially TV and Hollywood's depictions of female beauty.

Moms, I urge you to monitor what your children see and hear. We expose them to too much. If you're a mother of boys, please influence them about their views regarding women, how they view them, how they talk to them, how they treat them. It's far too easy for little boys to become men who think it's okay to treat women like objects, or like a set of body parts and nothing else. It's too easy for them to think it's okay to talk down to women or to catcall and objectify women. Raising boys who treat women with respect starts with you, and it also starts with monitoring what they see on TV.

The same goes for raising little girls, but in a different way. It only takes a couple of negative experiences to make a girl ashamed of her body, or make her think she has to be skinny to be beautiful. We need to offer positive experiences so our children can feel good about their bodies. Sometimes I wonder if the dance classes, football fields and baseball diamonds are cutting it.

So how does this play into how *you* feel about *your* body? What can we do as families to place a different value on our bodies? Running 5k races is a great place to start.

Yes, back to this.

First, it's a great bonding experience for your family. Second, it really isn't a team sport, so the whole family can have different goals, competing *together* rather than against each other. My husband and oldest son blaze to the finish, with my second oldest son not far behind, and my daughter and the younger three bringing up the rear with me. It doesn't really matter where we are in the race, only that we all finish.

I can't tell you how often I struggle near the end of the race, and then I see my husband and two boys at the finish line, cheering me on. Honestly, it's brought me to tears a few times. A year ago I'm sure they wouldn't have ever guessed I could run that far at all, much less without stopping to gasp for breath. It wasn't that they didn't believe in me—I didn't think I could do it either!

I'm sure you're sitting there thinking the same thing about yourself: running is for skinny people, for weird, preppy athletic people, it's for someone who needs a horde of zombies chasing them to be motivated to run. I get it, really I do. I can't tell you how many times I've joked that I don't run unless something is chasing me. Are there hungry bears? No? Then guess who's not running?

When I was a kid I always felt like I was going to die if I even tried to jog a block. Looking back on it though, it wasn't like anyone was really trying to teach me about running. I took dance classes several days a week and I swam like a fish, but I just never thought I could run. I'm not even sure why I thought that. I guess, in my mind, running had to do with aerodynamics and my big butt. I just wasn't ever going to get any speed going because I had too much dragging me down. I was partially right, but mostly I was wrong. I think we should teach every child that he or she *can* run, no matter what their body type, that running equals stamina, health, and energy. Plus, there's so much you can learn about yourself while running, because you have so much time to think.

I'm going to use my daughter as an example. I'm usually pretty private about my kids, but I know her story will inspire you, so I got her permission to share this. My daughter is ten years old and incredibly beautiful. She has one of those rare smiles that lights up a whole room. She's been a performer since she danced out of the womb. She was born a star, in every way, so you'd think a child like that would have lots of self confidence but, in reality, it's something she really struggles with. She's very hesitant to engage in most physical activity, so when we decided to do our first family 5k, she was the one who said she couldn't do it. The morning of the run she actually thought she was going to puke; she just didn't believe she could do it. Well, her brothers insisted she could, and promised to stay with her the whole way, so she took off with them.

Later on, when we caught up to her brothers, she was nowhere to be seen. We eventually found her walking with friends from school. She did end up running with me a little near the end, but she felt pretty defeated. So before the next race we did a few training runs with the kids at home, so they could practice. Our "block" around the farm is three and half miles, so it makes a pretty good practice course for a 5k. This time I got right behind her and told her how strong she was every single time she wanted to quit. I told her God gave her muscles and strength for a reason. I played her favorite songs and cheered her on. As always, it was just she and I dragging behind the big boys, but you could tell she was beginning to feel more confident.

The next race we entered was attended by three times the number people as our previous race. It was a qualifying event for the Boston marathon, so people came from all over to do it. These were *serious* runners we were with, so why the hell were we doing this?

My daughter took off like a rocket! I didn't see her again until we reached the end and I found her eating her fruit and drinking water at the finish line. That girl soared to the end and beat her best time by fifteen minutes! I can't even tell you how proud of her I was. It's amazing what having her family by her side did for her self-confidence. It's a huge boost when she hits a new personal best and then gets to celebrate with the family. She's still running, and the confidence she's gained from that experience shows in her dance classes as well. She holds herself with more confidence, and you can see she has more respect for her body.

Let's tell our kids how strong they are, *show* them how strong they are, and then stand back and watch how far they can go with it. You'll be surprised!

Inspire each other.

Do healthy, challenging activities together as a family. There's no better way to spend time together. It certainly beats sitting on your butt watching TV!

I'm talking to you specifically, Mama, because I'm hearing you say your husband wouldn't do this with you, or that your kids would cry and complain the whole time, or that you'd embarrass them just by going out in your gym clothes. Stop that negative bullshit RIGHT NOW! Ain't nobody got time for that! You aren't going to get this time back, so don't waste it lying to yourself. Your body is able to walk, crawl, run, jog, or wog to the finish line. It might take you a solid hour, and that is totally fine. Maybe your husband won't join you, or maybe he'll tell you it's a total waste of time and money. Fine!

Let him think that. But when you come home with your participant's T-shirt, looking all healthy and hot, and he might be inspired to try it with you next time. There's pride in wearing a shirt you can only get by running a 5k. You can't buy it; you can't get it in stores or on Amazon. You only get that shirt by running the race. That shirt? It's a point of pride. Your kids will notice, I promise you. They'll say "Hey, Mom, can you sign me up for the next one?"

I'm not a doctor, and I'm not a life coach, but I *am* a mother of six, so I think I have a pretty firm grasp on kids and family life. I know it's hard, but I also know our nation is full of physically, mentally, and emotionally unhealthy children. It's up to us as parents to change the status quo, for them, for ourselves, and for future generations. Change starts at home.

The idea of "running with your tribe" has serious merit; even a hundred years ago families worked, played, and explored together in a way we simply don't do anymore, at any level. Life was active. If you wanted something, you worked for it. Our day-to-day lives are so dominated by convenience and ease that if it isn't right in the palm of our hands we can't be bothered to make the effort, and our kids are picking up on that. We've become complacent and lazy as a culture. I'm sorry if that's offensive, but I'm just being honest, and I'm including myself in this.

Have you ever seen the Pixar film *WALL-E*? Those giant slobs incapable of walking on their own two feet? That will be us in a few generations if we don't start making changes. We are becoming less and less physically active as a culture; because every new device and piece of technology is aimed at making everything easier, more convenient, requiring less work and less effort. Even when I watch my kids play soccer I find myself thinking about how little effort so many kids are willing to put in. Unless the coach is yelling at them to run, they're standing around idle, or even sitting down.

So, I'm challenging them on it now. I'm challenging myself. I'm challenging you and your family. I'm reaching out to all you ladies between twenty and fifty years old who are my core readership. You've really poured your hearts out to me about your struggles with weight. I know how hard it is. I know it seems hopeless. I know what I'm asking of you right now feels utterly daunting. You feel like you've failed before you've even begun.

You haven't!

You can do this!

Put the book down, *right now*, and get on your gym clothes.

…I'll wait.

Still waiting…..

I'm not even kidding about this. Get those gym clothes on! Whatever you've got that even remotely resembles workout clothes, get 'em on!

I want you to stand in front of the mirror and say this out loud.

Yes, this again.

Say it like you really mean it. Say it for yourself, and for your kiddos.

They need a strong, healthy mama; they deserve it! They, and you, deserve the best version of you!

So say it with me, one more time, with bone-deep conviction:

"God meant for my body to be healthy and strong.

I am worth the time it will take to make myself stronger and healthier.

It won't be easy, but it will be worth it.

Yes, it's okay to do this for those who love me as well, but this is for me.

I was beautiful then, I am beautiful now, and I will be beautiful tomorrow.

I can do this.

I can do this despite feeling like I can't, or that I've been told I can't.

My body is beautiful at any size.

My body is going to be unstoppable when I'm healthier and stronger, so watch out!

Nothing will define me.

Nothing will stop me.

I can do this!"

Now I want you to run around your block. One block. I don't care if you have to stop and walk for a while.

You aren't even allowed to turn the page until you've run that one block. I mean it! I'm from Detroit and I will kick your ass if you don't run around that block. Don't make me show up at your house. I will.

I'll be right here when you get back.

Ready…set…go!

Race Day pro tip: Make sure to pack snacks and extra water. A healthy breakfast of egg whites and toast with some turkey bacon or sausage or some oatmeal is my go-to pre-race breakfast.

Chapter 17

LET'S TALK RUNNING GEAR!

NOW WE GET TO TALK ABOUT ONE OF MY VERY FAVORITE PARTS of running: getting suited up! Let me start by saying you really don't *need* anything special to run, not even shoes—there are even whole groups dedicated to running barefoot! I don't really advise that unless you're seriously committed to running, though. You can buy some cheap shoes at Wal-Mart or Target, if you are on a budget; I'm currently in love with my size thirteen NYC edition ASICS Gel Nimbus 17s I got from Amazon for a steal of a deal. They feel like heaven on my feet and are so easy on my knees.

That being said, when I started this journey I really wanted to discover what I liked to wear, and what worked best for my body, so I tried countless different brands and styles. When you're bigger it can be hard to find clothes you feel comfortable working out in and that fit well, so I applaud a lot of the big-box stores and mall clothing lines for adding these items in their stores.

I like to browse Amazon and compare prices to what is available in the stores—you'd be surprised how much of a price difference you might find on certain items. Old Navy also has a much better sizing selection online than in stores; I've found things up to a 4x on Old

Navy's website, and those are usually hard to find in a retail store at a decent price. I also really, *really* like the Calia by Carrie Underwood workout clothes. They're higher in price but the quality is great, and they also have plus sizes.

We have a small, local running store in town that we really love. Employees at your local running store have a wealth of knowledge on anything from fitting a good running bra to testing your feet for which shoe fits best, so make sure you check yours out if you have one local.

Running as a big girl can add some additional challenges. When I first started running I noticed my body was fighting me in certain areas. Now, I'm going to get a bit personal here, but I'm sure some ladies reading this will find this information helpful, so I'm not holding anything back. I've got a big chest, butt, and thighs so I knew, after running for a few weeks, that I would need extra support in those areas. As I continued to run I lost weight and I noticed my belly skin getting a bit looser, so it was easy to see I needed some help there, too. This is totally normal and okay!

Wearing support garments when you run will help you run longer, farther, and faster. You have to know and understand your body—this might be an issue for you, and it might not, it just depends on your body. You may start with no hanging skin and then find that with exercise and weight loss you need to tuck and compress in some places. I believe in doing anything necessary to be comfortable while exercising.

A few months ago I started testing different types of clothing to see what I felt worked best. In terms of sports bras, I think you really should invest in a good one if you've got a larger chest. If you're a B cup it might not be a problem, but if you're a DD, you're really going to want to strap those puppies down tight. I like Panache or

Under Armor bras, sized down a little so I'm absolutely sure nothing is gonna pop out. Yes, these are a bit expensive, but this is something worth investing in. You don't want to give yourself a black eye while running.

Another thing that's really helped me is a Squeem tummy supporter, and I also like the Sweet Sweat brand. I wear them over a tank or running shirt and it helps me keep my stomach in place while I'm running. Now, I'm not sure it would work for everyone but, after being pregnant so many times, having that extra stomach support is great—it actually helps me run faster.

I also make sure to wear high quality compression tights or pants, and now I'm often running with wraps around my thighs as well. Again, all this does is give me extra support and it makes me more aerodynamic. If you've lost a lot of weight, these things can really help, so don't be afraid to try them. I think it's much better to invest in good support garments than to just quit running because your skin is in the way. This is nothing to be embarrassed about! Your body is getting lean, mean, strong, and sassy; so don't let anything hold you back, literally or figuratively.

I also think you need music. If you're walking or wogging with a friend, then this might not be as important. I know, for me, when Jack and I run together he ends up way ahead and then my mind starts to wander, so music helps me to keep going; I've actually plotted out two books while running! It's a great time for inspiration, prayer, focus, and meditation. These things are important, so why not have a good soundtrack to go with them?

There are some amazing playlists out there—I'm a pretty lazy person when it comes to making my own playlists, so I usually just buy those cheesy "workout mixes" and run to those. Hip Hop is awesome to run to—check out my playlist at the end of the book for some of my favorites. My husband prefers to listen to death metal when he runs, but he's a weird one. Just find something you like and get moving!

When I first started running I wanted those cute in-ear buds I saw everyone wearing at the races but, guess what? They just didn't work for me. I would be running and then one would literally fly out of my ear. I must have odd shaped ears or something, because I would put them in and go on my merry way, and then *bam*, they'd fly out again. I was worried one was going to hit some other poor runner in the eye.

I use some pretty sweet Beats By Dre when I write but they have a cord that gets in the way when I'm running, so finally, after months of headphone drama, I broke down and bought some wireless over-ear Beats that stay on my head and sound amazing. Yes, they're pricy, but *dude*, I'm not scrambling all over the road trying to find those stupid buds that kept shooting out of my ears. It was so worth it!

You may feel a bit self-conscious when you run outside the first few times. It's weird, because I only feel that way in high traffic situations, like suddenly there's a bunch of cars zipping past, and I freak out a tiny bit. They're staring at me! Do I look okay? This is totally normal, so if you have the funds, go and get a few sets of exercise clothes you feel sexy in. I personally love pink and other bright colors, so I have a whole bunch of pink running gear—it makes me feel badass and sexy—and it gives me a bit of comfort in the knowledge that drivers will see me when they drive down our main road where I run; it's pretty hard to miss a six-foot-tall lady in bright pink from head to toe.

Another item I stumbled upon and fell in love with was the running skirt or tutu. These skirts are so darn cute and so comfortable to run in! When it's warm out you'll see me running in a super cute, limited edition Cupcake running skirt. Mine even has pockets! It doesn't ride up and will keep you cool when you walk, wog or jog. They also hide any extra movement you might have in the rear, if you have a bit of junk going on in your trunk.

I really think it's the little things that keep you going. Consider making this running skirt a reward for meeting a goal or besting your previous record. They come in all sizes, colors, and shapes, so I'm sure you'll find one you like. If you need help picking one out, just let me know, because I love shopping for this stuff!

I also sweat a *lot,* so I wear a lot of fun headbands that keep my hair and sweat from being all in my face. This stuff will make you feel sporty and super cute! A word of caution, though: you should *NOT* do crazy makeup on a race day. It's only going to stay on your face for about two seconds, and then it'll be running down your face and stinging your eyes and getting in your mouth and it'll taste nasty and you'll look like a bedraggled raccoon, so no to the make-up. However, I do make sure my nails are painted, and I always wear sunscreen and some lip-gloss.

If you're running in the cold like I am *ALL THE TIME*, then make sure to keep some lip balm or gloss with you—good running pants will have a little pocket you can stick it in. I love my Graced By Grit running jacket because it also has awesome arm pockets for my phone and other things I might bring with me, and you can also get some really cheap running belts that will hold your phone, keys, gloss etc. Just don't forget to remove your belongings before you wash your stinky running clothes!

I also want to talk a bit about running tech. There are so many awesome wrist gadgets on the market that I think it's important to touch on this topic for a moment. I've tested the FitBit, Garmin and the Apple Watch while I've been running. For me, it's a toss up between the FitBit and Garmin wearables. Both of them have a heart rate monitor, and I also like their social media notifications.

All of these options have great apps that will track your progress and help motivate you on a daily basis, and you can even challenge your family and friends, especially with the Garmin. The Apple Watch is awesome if you have the budget for it—I've actually called my husband from my watch while running. It's great for emergencies too, like the time a wheel busted off the jogging stroller and Jack was a mile ahead of me.

We really like Apple products in our family: we all work on Macs, even the kids, and neither Jack nor I can go anywhere without our big iPhone 6 Plus. The Apple Watch health app is really cool because it sort of learns your habits and challenges you to push harder. It's sort of like having a personal trainer on your wrist—my watch will prompt me to get up and move every hour, which actually does make me think about standing up and moving around when I've been on my butt working for too long. It always pushes me to work out harder and longer, and prompts me to beat my last time.

The other really cool thing we've found is a weigh scale that connects to our health apps; it's nice to be able to see a graph of your health stats all in one place, right on your cell phone. I've seen these scales priced from between $50 and $200, so if this is something that might really help you, go for it!

In no way are any of these things necessary, but they are cool and they provide added incentives. Knowing the cycle of your body and being able to see each morning if those pesky weight fluctuations are muscle, water, or hormone cycles is useful knowledge to have. Because we waste so much time guessing, having the real info in the palm of your hand can be a relief and a blessing.

Just don't become obsessed with the numbers. Your body needs grace and time.

Pro Tip: When looking for shoes it's a great idea to get fitted at your local running shop. Many of them will have you step on a machine that can figure out which particular shoe will be best for you. You'll need a half to full size larger than your normal sneaker for running, so it's a good idea to be professionally fitted. Get the pink, orange, or purple ones! Stand out in the crowd!

Chapter 18

RUNNING FUN VS RUNNING FAR!

So, you just finished your first 5k and now you think you want to do a full marathon. Let's put on the brakes for a moment—I'm not at all against long distance running, and I'm not going to tell you not to do it, but I am going to offer a word of warning. I want this to be fun for you and your whole family. I want this to become a part of your lifestyle. Wouldn't it be cool to pick a vacation destination because there's a fun themed 5k or 10k race, or maybe your whole family did your local Turkey Trot every Thanksgiving? That's what I hope you do with this. I want you to get moving. I want running to become something you look forward to, maybe even crave.

What I don't want is for it to become a pressure for you, or to cause injury.

Long distance running isn't for everyone—I get that. I think a fun 5k or 10k is healthy and can be super fun for the whole family. You aren't taxing your body too hard, you can walk if you have to, and you can have a great time while getting in some good exercise.

Remember, we're looking for *long-term* health and moderation. We want to give your body time to heal, recover, and strengthen. Please continue to see your doctor during this time and take it easy.

If you want to run a marathon next year, then let's get you healthy and as strong as possible first, because a marathon is no joke. Even a 10k is something to work up to gradually. There's a lot of evidence that says that the more quickly we jump head first into things, the less likely we are to stick with them.

So my challenge to you for this first year as a runner—or for those of you getting back to running after being away from it—is to do four races max, maybe one 5k each quarter. Pick some really fun ones so you can laugh a lot and enjoy yourself. Make this about celebrating your body and your health, which is what this is really all about. The truth is, running is going to become addictive. Once you get started, you're really going to love it. I want you walking, running, jogging, or wogging three to four times a week for about thirty minutes. I think that is really all you need.

I only want about an hour and a half each week from you. And since I'm so nice, I'm even going to allow you one day of whatever kind of exercise you want—Zumba, baseball, half an hour of sex are all great!

This might sound too easy but, actually, it really is just that simple. You have a total of 168 hours in your week; so just give me one and a half hours of fun, physical movement. You should enjoy your life, so I want you to have fun with this. If it's a little hard sometimes and you hate me while you're running, that's fine. I'm okay with you hating me as long as you're moving. But you hating it so much you never do it again, that I'm not okay with! I want you to be physically active for the rest of your life. I want you on your feet using the beautiful body God gave you. There are some weeks I even count dancing in my kitchen as my workout. Kitchen dancing is so much fun, and it's something the whole family can do together, too.

What, you don't kitchen dance? Well, you should totally start.

Pro tip: wine helps.

If you're at the point where you're still unable to walk, run, or wog a 5k, don't beat yourself up, or injure yourself trying. You might need a few extra months of training, and that's fine too! You'll get there! Remember, my first 5k was almost my funeral! Just keep challenging yourself in positive ways. You can always do short bursts of fast walking or wogging and then go back to walking. You *will* get to that 5k, just keep going.

So, I'll stop proselytizing for a minute and ask you a few simple questions: What's going to be your first 5k? Your second? Where would you like to run? Who would you like to run with? Who could you inspire with your running? Who could you run in memory, or in honor of?

These are things I really want you to think about. Everything we're doing is supposed to be fun, and all about you. This isn't a one-size-fits-all program—this is *your* plan for *your* health, so there are no boundaries, no limits, and no minimum requirements. Give yourself time to heal and strengthen, so you can really soar! Once we get you going, there will be no stopping you! Just have fun. Keep pushing yourself and enjoy the ride. I'm already proud of the things you're going to accomplish.

If you find yourself in need of support on your journey to health, please know you can contact me on Facebook. I've set up a group called BIG GIRLS DO IT RUNNING on Facebook that is there to motivate and inspire you, and to answer any questions you may have. Please feel free to join us, because you are *not* in this alone. This is a revolution of health and wellness. All are welcome!

Pro tip: It's a great idea to keep a journal to record your journey to health and wellness. Track your progress, set new goals, and note the details when you reach a goal, or set a new record. You will feel so good about yourself when you read back on your early entries and realize how far you have come.

Chapter 19

CHAFING, RUNNER'S ITCH, AND STUFF I PROBABLY SHOULDN'T MENTION

"Runner's itch sucks." – Jasinda Wilder

I DON'T WANT TO DISCOURAGE YOU IN ANY WAY WHEN IT COMES TO being more active. Getting your body moving and building up strength and endurance is awesome! Remember weeks ago when it was difficult to even get up the stairs? It's a breeze now, right?

I do want to touch on some of the possibly not so good things that might crop up for you. If you're a bigger girl—or guy—you might encounter some chafing and rubbing issues, particularly on your thighs. Remember when I talked about having the right garments? Well, it really is very important. If you're wearing some old, ratty gym shorts you borrowed from your husband, it's only going to make chafing and rubbing worse. Wearing some good compression tights or support pants will help a lot. You can also try powder or lotions to keep any problem areas dry or lubricated as needed.

In my experience, running in the cold it seems to make the itching and chafing worse, so I'm a *huge* fan of coconut oil. I also really like the Naturewell Extra Virgin Coconut Oil Moisturizing Cream…

that stuff is actual magic for your skin. I rub some into my skin before I put my tights, and it really helps alleviate the effects of chafing.

You also may want to have lots of lubrication under your bra if you're going to be wogging or jogging. You may encounter some pretty serious redness and rubbing where the bra straps touch your skin, so don't be afraid to use some oil or lotion in those areas too—the last thing you want is scratching or chafing all over the girls.

I've noticed my bra seems to get tighter as I run, and I have no clue why. Maybe my skin expands? I don't know. I'm sure there's a scientific explanation for it, but all I know is that it happens. If you're going to be running a long distance—anything over three miles, for me—I would suggest loosening the straps a little. I once tried to adjust my bra while running and that was a big mistake; the driver of a big truck that was going down the street saw me and, well, I can tell you how well *that* went. It may even be worth a trial run if the bra is new, since it's not fun to get half way through your run only to find yourself fighting tears because your bra is digging into your skin somewhere. My advice is to spend some money on a good sports bra. The girls need your support.

Winter running isn't for the weak up here in northern Michigan. When we first started running this winter I developed a crazy itch—it felt as if my legs were on fire and tiny ants were having a dance party on them. I finally talked to my doctor and she said there's an actual thing called "runner's itch" which can cause your body to itch like mad. She said that, basically, my body was becoming allergic to exercise! Isn't that just hilarious? Ha…ha? Yeah, *not* so funny.

After the appointment I did a bit more investigation and discovered it's very common to have an allergy-type reaction to running, depending on the environment. The extreme cold was already making my skin dry, and the running was just aggravating the condition.

If this does happen to you, don't freak out. It isn't ants, bugs, or a deadly flesh-eating virus. If I survived runner's itch, you can too. Just don't do what I did one time. I went for a run, took a shower, forgot to put on lotion, and then put on tights, and then tried to sit still for a three-hour movie date with my husband. I do NOT suggest that… *at all.*

I have another important PSA I should probably put out there. Are you ready for it? Gosh, it's so embarrassing that I'm not sure I can type it!

Running makes you poop!

I didn't even know about this until I decided to take a long run with my husband, only to find myself making a mad dash for the toilet as soon as we got home. Don't worry though; you *probably* won't poop your pants. I mean, you might, and I'm sure it will happen to someone, but hopefully it won't happen to you. Fingers crossed. (I'm likely just giving you more reasons not to run, but it's just I want to make sure you're fully informed before you start. The best surprise is no surprise.)

Running really is amazing, once you get started. I really, truly, deeply believe you're going to love it…just get ready to shit your brains out afterward. The great thing is that pooping is good for you. A healthy body and a healthy metabolism will promote regular, healthy bowel movements. Just know going in that it's totally normal and you shouldn't be embarrassed.

The final thing I want to cover in this chapter is stinking. I mean, since we talked about pooping, we may as well talk about body odor, too. When we first started on our health journey, I switched to a more natural deodorant. I'd tried them before and never had much luck, but since I was sweating and working out I decided now was a good time to test a few more out; I wanted to minimize my body odor in a more natural way. I tried a few different products but none of them would go on well or stay on, and if they did they didn't minimize the smell very well.

I finally found a lavender-scented deodorant I really liked, but it wouldn't last very long. And then, while browsing our local farm co-op, I spotted a few natural body odor sprays and tried a few of those, but they didn't last very long either. I was getting frustrated. Then, one morning, out of sheer exhaustion and caffeine-deprived desperation, I put them both on and guess what? I had forty-eight hours without stinking! No joke! Something about layering the stick and the spray gave me some superhuman B.O. coverage. Now that's all I use, and even Jack is doing the same thing. There were a few days where I had some weird detox thing, but now I almost never have any body odor, even after a long run or workout session.

Jack and I will do kettlebell workouts together once in a while, and I always sweat so much more during those sessions. I'm always so surprised that I never need to worry about body odor. I'm a human daisy!

I do think it's worth looking for deodorant products that are more natural, and there are many good products out there these days. Jack even found one he likes that makes him smell like "the woods". I think it's a guy thing.

Chapter 20

SUPPLEMENTS, BEAUTY AND FASHION, OH MY!

My maternal grandmother didn't see a doctor from the time she had my uncle at forty years old until the day she died at eighty-five. She didn't believe doctors had any medicine for her that she couldn't find at the health store. I thought she was crazy—I mean, I loved her dearly but I think there's a middle ground between modern medicine and simply eating well and taking supplements. I don't take a ton of supplements, but I do think there are a few worth taking to promote overall good health.

- You need a good multivitamin. Make sure if you choose a chewable that has no added sugar. My kids love the Smarty Pants No Sugar Added with Fiber. Lots of bang for your buck.
- I put integral collagen and MTC oil in my coffee each morning. The MTC oil helps with my blood and nutritional deficiency, and collagen is wonderful for your complexion, among other benefits. I haven't had a single breakout or skin issue since I started taking it. It also helps promote healthy lashes, nails and hair!
- I also put Bragg Apple Cider vinegar in my morning LaCroix. It's really helped me curb sugar cravings, and it also has many

other health benefits: prevents stomach illness, dissolves kidney stones, regulates PH balance and blood pressure, lowers glucose levels, and provides relief from nausea, heart burn, acid reflux, asthma, allergies, and gout, migraines, sinus pressure and infections, inflammation, bug bites, rash, warts and acne! Just mix it into water with lemon and drink it in the morning. Why would you pass up all those health benefits?

- Vitamin C. I use it on my face. I know it sounds gross, but go check out the Amazon reviews for the Foxbrim brand (I really like that whole line of products, so check them out), and you'll find that huge numbers of people are seeing some great results from it. I swear, the day I turned 35 my face started looking older. Not that aging really bothers me, but I want to take care of my skin, so I use a good face lotion and vitamin C, and people have said they have noticed a glow. I'm a mom of six, I'll take whatever I can get!

- Probiotics are important. Why? They help with your immunity, assist with bowel issues, and will also help keep good bacteria in your body. Take a probiotic especially during the detox phase to make sure the good stuff is staying in and all the bad stuff is going out!

- I take Cod Liver Oil and Vitamin D every day. It helps with my immunity, inflammation, and nutritional issues, and they've also been shown to help with depression. As always, talk to your doctor about your vitamin and supplement needs.

- Getting enough fiber is vital. My little boys had terrible issues with constipation, so I make sure everyone stays regular with a fiber supplement—I use PGX Fiber by Webber Naturals. We also use a powder for the kids that's totally invisible and tasteless, made by Renew Life. It's great because they don't even know they're getting it. It is also available on Amazon. Fiber is so, *so* important for a healthy diet, but don't overdo it…you don't want to poop lava.

- Bathe and shower with Epsom salts. Release those yucky toxins! I buy giant bags from Amazon and add some coconut oil to make a salt scrub. You can also add a bit of an essential oil and fancy it up a notch—works as a scrub or a soak.

You'll start seeing changes almost overnight. Some weeks the changes will be numeric and you'll see the pounds melt away. Other weeks you'll go down a clothing size, but your weight will stay the same. My mother, several friends, and a beta testing group will all tell you that if you do everything I'm laying out for you in this book you'll start dropping excess weight immediately.

For me this was both a blessing and a curse. Most of you probably know that over the past three years I was traveling several weeks each month for book tours, speaking events, and signings. I'd built up a pretty kick-ass wardrobe—in size twenty-two. I'd been wearing so much maternity clothing over the years that those items were extra special to me. Alas, I shrunk from a twenty-two to a size eighteen in the blink of an eye, and then down to a fourteen! These changes happened over a matter of months. None of my clothes fit anymore!

So, what do we do about clothes that no longer fit? We give them away. I found lots of special ladies to bless with those clothes—some were even brought to tears. You can also find a consignment or resale store where you can swap or donate clothes. It's a very real possibility that you won't be wearing new clothes for very long. I suggest going for leggings, or anything with some stretch to it. Also, there are fun online boutiques like The Zig Zag Stripe and Lu La Roe that have been a huge blessing for me as I constantly change sizes. They have one-size-fits-most clothing, which will stretch and shrink with you, so I can hold on to my new items for a little longer. It's just so much more economical as you don't really know where you're going to end up size-wise, so try to buy on the smaller size and wear those clothes as long as you can. It's a good problem to have.

I believe you need to find a goal outfit. I know I've already said it isn't about the numbers, and I just want to reiterate that. It's not about the numbers on the scale, or the numbers on the tag! It's about feeling good and looking good, so find something in your closet that's a little tight, something you've wanted to wear but couldn't because it's been too small. Maybe it's even your wedding dress, or a sexy little black dress from college. Whatever it is, pick something that will motivate you on your journey to wellness, something that shows where you came from and where you're headed. Take that dress or outfit out of your closet and put it somewhere where you can see it all the time.

You're worth it! Don't let that goal out of sight.

You're going to be wearing that outfit before you know it!

Chapter 21

THE WILDER WAY FOR THE PREGNANT MAMA

I WAS HALFWAY THOUGH MY MOST RECENT PREGNANCY WHEN WE started making health changes. My doctor was thrilled with what I was doing and the positive effects it was having on my pregnancy. It's critical that you discuss what's best for you with your doctor. I do know whole foods free of chemicals and additives are going to be wonderful for you and the baby, and that stabilizing your blood sugars and insulin levels will help prevent gestational diabetes, which is something so many women deal with during pregnancy.

Be sure that if you do lose weight you discuss the weight loss with your doctor; my OB felt that as long as the baby was measuring normal my weight loss was a good thing. Your OB might not want you to lose too much weight during the pregnancy, depending on where you were before conception. You can always eat more good carbs for extra energy, and there's nothing wrong with eating any good, nutritious, whole foods while pregnant.

Running during pregnancy isn't something I personally would want to do, but some women do it. Again, this is something you should talk to your doctor about. I didn't start running until Ree was about two months old. By that time I didn't feel like a total zombie, and I actually wanted to get out there and move. I did walk a lot when I was pregnant with her, and unless you have some issue or condition during your pregnancy I would think most doctors would be totally fine with the idea of you walking three or four times a week, even pretty far into your pregnancy.

Actually, the closer we got to my due date the more we walked. I've always had very long and complicated deliveries, and the only thing that was different with Ree was that my health and eating habits had changed drastically in comparison to my other pregnancies and deliveries. I believe being more physically fit at the end of my pregnancy made my delivery so much easier.

The awesome thing about pregnancy is that it will help you tune into your body in a way you might not when you aren't pregnant. I'm so grateful that my pregnancy and baby Ree helped me finally understand what was going on with my blood sugar. I was able to make much-needed changes to my health—my body was demanding these changes, and I finally *had* to listen. I've never in my life craved bacon and eggs like I did when I was pregnant: my body needed fat and protein for the baby, and those cravings were my body's way of informing me.

If you are pregnant, I suggest keeping a journal to write down what you're experiencing—this is important information that you might want to refer to in the future. Pregnancy is an illuminating time. I really wish I'd kept better records of my health during my first two pregnancies, as it would be great to compare the differences.

I recently watched a video about infants becoming obese; the doctors said they believe the health of the mother during pregnancy was the causal factor in the strange phenomenon. The baby's glucose levels are being set in the womb and the baby will start demanding similar levels after delivery. The nutritionist in the video said the best way to prevent this decline in babies' health is to advocate for prevention of obesity in the mother prior to her childbearing years.

As women go from being adolescents to teenagers and adults, it's important they focus on their health for the wellbeing of their future children. This struck me so hard: I have a 10 year old daughter, and I want to teach her to be healthy and strong *now*, while she's young enough to make it a lifestyle. Me teaching her healthy living habits won't just affect her, but it will also affect my future grandchildren and *their* children.

The last thirty years of American culture has had drastic affects on us, and not necessarily for the better. Now is the time for us to start showing our kids a better way to eat, a better way to view their bodies. I'm not talking about size or numbers; I'm talking about positive nutrition and strength.

If you're a mom, pregnant, or thinking about becoming pregnant, I urge you to take a look at the quick-start guide at the back of my book, and talk about healthy eating with your doctor. The food we eat while pregnant has a massive, long-lasting impact on our children as they develop in utero and as they grow after birth. Motherhood is both an honor and a responsibility, one we *have* to take seriously. I know this might sound like a lot to think about, especially if this is your first child, but you won't get this time back. Being a mother is the greatest and most difficult job you'll ever have; if you focus on your health first, your child will be better for it in the long run. Get healthy now, mama. Make it a priority! Kids keep you on your toes, and sometimes bring you to your knees, so you're going to need every healthy molecule and burst of energy you can find!

Chapter 22

YOU FINISHED THE BOOK...NOW WHAT?

"The most difficult thing is the decision to act, the rest is merely tenacity." – Amelia Earhart

Now that you've reached this point in the book I hope you've found it both educational and fun to read; I know I really enjoyed the process of writing it. Honestly, though, this book isn't about me, it's all about *you*.

What follows is The Wilder Way, an eight-week health plan and 25 of my favorite family recipes. You might not even get to those, you might close the book right now and never take a step toward improving your health; you may be thinking it's too hard, or it won't work for you, or that you're not worth the time and effort. I disagree. I don't think there's anything else *more* important than your health, and by health I mean everything—your body, spirit and mind.

Yes, I'm gonna get all hippie and metaphysical on you. You aren't just the sum of your parts—you are an amazing woman designed to be healthy, strong, and bold. Ponder all the times you've been excited about something only to fail—I get it, I've been there a thousand times myself, from that first time I put my Teen Steam dance video in my VCR to the last time I tried a fancy new diet. Nothing ever worked for me. So I understand the fear all too well—I know that fear far too intimately.

Stay strong; *this* will work, I promise.

I want you to close your eyes and imagine yourself healthy and fit. What that looks like is different for everyone. I know what that looks like for me: I want this port out of my chest; I want to finish a 10k in an hour and fifteen minutes; I want my belly to be full of healthy fuel, and my muscles to be beautiful and strong; I don't want to worry about diabetes looming; I don't want to be nutritionally deficient; I want to look *damn* good in my size twelve dress and sexy heels. That's what health looks like to me, and for the first time in my life, I feel *so* close to having just that. I've got it within my grasp, ladies. I'm almost there! And you can be, too.

Look at the cover of this book; do I look healthy and happy to you? Through all the trials and tribulations, through all the false starts and failures, I've learned that my body *does* work. Right now, my body's fat mass is within a healthy range for the first time in my life! My legs are strong. I've got powerful biceps. My back doesn't hurt anymore.

What about you? What's your story? What's your final goal, and how are you going to make that vision in your head become a reality?

All you need is eight weeks to change your life; I don't think eight weeks is a long time, do you? Yes, there are things that might be difficult in those weeks. In fact I'm pretty sure people will send me nasty emails around week five. I'm okay with that! You can even email Jack about how horrible I am for putting you through this, but I know that by week eight, I'll be getting an equally awesome apology email. One that says your inflammation is now gone, that you final-ly have a normal blood sugar level, and maybe there will even be a photo of your face looking years younger. You'll tell me that not only did you lose weight but also, for the first time in your life, you have self-confidence and strength and you feel sexy in your skin.

I want those things for you! I want you to learn what I've learned on this journey: most of us weren't born with something wrong with us. Most of us aren't genetically challenged. We don't lack will power, we don't need to cut ourselves open and remove portions of our intestines, we don't need to sleeve, band, or starve ourselves to be healthy.

It's about food combinations. It's about moving. It's about kicking sugar to the curb and never looking back.

Please believe me when I say that if this hot mess mother of six can do it, you can too. I know it!

What I would love for you to do is read through the start-up plan and the recipes that follow—all the way to the very end—and then I want you to take some time and think about why you want this. Why is this your moment? Why are you finally done with all the diets, the workout fads, and gimmicks. Why is *now* the moment when true health is going to be your goal?

Before I even started writing this book, I knew it would be the most important book I ever wrote. I feel a responsibility, an obligation, to use my story to help people. Even if only a few people pick it up, I know I can change those lives forever. I have the ability to reach people who would *never* pick up a health book unless it was written by me. What an honor! If you've never read any other health or fitness book before, then you picked the right one! This is going to be a system you can live with, and it will allow you to enjoy life as never before.

Take it one day at a time, one meal at a time. Stick with me even when it gets hard, even when you see the scale creep up during the challenge weeks. It's okay, it happens, and it will come back down. Give your body grace and time—you deserve that. Your body needs time to heal from the lifetime of damage that sugar and chemicals and refined carbs have done to it. Detox is a gift to your body, but you have to give it time.

If I could talk to you right now, I would ask which race will be your first—I'm so excited for you to cross that finish line! I can see it in my head, and it makes me want to cry for you, for *all* of us who never thought we were capable of running, for those of us who never believed our bodies could cross a finish line without being dragged across by paramedics. You—yes *YOU*—will finish that race, and it will be glorious.

Then I would tell you to take this one week at a time. Follow the plan I've laid out. Yes, you could take a short cut, but it won't do any good in the long run. This is four weeks of detox and four weeks of learning how to create your meals; that time is crucial, so don't skip it.

The last thing I would do is tell you this is a journey you should enjoy. The year or two it will take to transform your health is a blessing. How many people will you inspire? How many lives will be changed watching you take control over your health and your life? Just remember, I'm going to be here cheering you on the whole way! I hope you connect with me on social media and share your progress—I can't wait to watch you run wild!

Please remember to consult with your doctor before starting any new health plan. If you are already being treated for diabetes or blood pressure, talking with your doctor regularly is very important.

PART 4

The Wilder Way

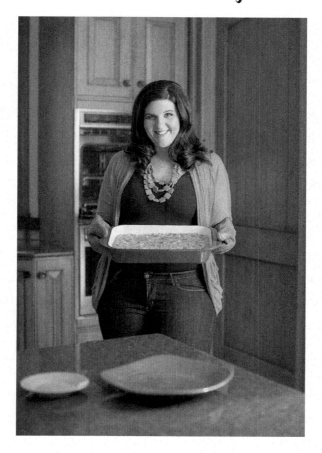

MY 8-WEEK GET-STARTED GUIDE

WELCOME!

   I am so glad you're here.

   This is the first step on the journey to reset your health. If you've been feeling tired, depressed, fat, and lazy, leave that all behind and get ready for one hell of a *WILD* ride. Don't think about other plans you've tried in the past, this one is totally different. We're going to get your body in fighting shape and moving like a warrior in just 8 weeks.

   When I first began eating in this new way, I would either pull back on my carbs or my fats depending on my needs for the meal; I was trying to replicate the way my body naturally wanted to eat when I was pregnant with my last child. After that pregnancy, and when I was going to have a workout day, I would do a meal or two with carbs for more energy and pull back on the fats for those meals. It was just the easiest way for me to do it—I didn't have to count anything and there were no carb caps or measuring or portions to worry about. Just mixing things up kept my body guessing and then adding in regular exercise was really all I needed to get my body in better health.

When my beta group began testing this 8-week plan, the carbs and fats got a bit confusing to them, so I told them it seemed black and white to me—and the idea of the black and white plates that you will read more about coming up emerged from there.

For black plates, the idea is to reduce or eliminate carbs, and for white plates carbs are included but fats are reduced. Protein is always the number one focus, regardless of plate color.

This 8-week plan is set up to gradually reduce your dependency on sugar in a slow, sustained detox, and then slowly ease you into an easy carb cycling lifestyle. This is NOT a diet; this is a new way of life, a new way of eating, and a new way of thinking about food. Try to take it one week at a time and don't overwhelm yourself. Slow and steady wins the race.

You can do this! How do I know? Because if I can do it, anyone can.

On your mark, get set…

GO!

WEEK 1

WEEK 1 CHALLENGE

This is a slow and steady, from-the-inside-out approach. No quick fixes. We're retraining your body and mind, and that takes time. I don't want you to ever feel frustrated or deprived. I've made these challenges doable for any fitness level, age, or overall health condition.

The first step is to detox your body from the biggest culprits behind the majority of health issues:

First, no sugar at breakfast. None. Focus on protein-rich foods, and completely cut out all sugar before noon. There are sixty-one names for sugar, so please make sure nothing you eat has it hidden in the ingredients. Yes, honey and agave are sugar. You can use stevia as a sweetener—my favorite brands are Pyure and Swerve. You can get them at the grocery store or on Amazon. Try eggs, bacon (remember, fats *ARE* your friend), oatmeal, yogurt (Greek without any added sugar), cottage cheese, toasted Ezekiel brand bread, or cereal with unsweetened almond milk. Berries are great too, so you can load up on those for some natural sweetness. Coffee can be creamed with half and half or heavy whipping cream.

Second, find a 5k to run in the next six months. There are tons of great races out there, so I'm positive you can find one near you. Ask, beg, or coerce a friend or family member to do it with you. If you have kids, I encourage you to include them too—a 5K is fun, healthy, and a great motivator to get moving. Walk if you're not there yet. Or you can try wogging. A 5K is three point one miles from start to finish, so it will take you about an hour, max. You don't even need to start training right now, just commit to running one 5K in your near future. You are *going* to cross a finish line!

WEEK 1 ENCOURAGEMENT

I've studied my ass off trying to figure out why so many of us struggle with excess weight and poor health. I think we fail because we are set up to fail. Why can some people eat whatever they want yet never gain weight, while some of us eat normal amounts and still gain weight? Why won't our bodies work right?

Some of us have had our metabolism literally shut down because of what's being put in our food. We've been eating food we think is healthy, food we're being *told* is healthy, but it's killing us, causing illnesses like diabetes and cancer.

Here's the deal—your current health and weight have nothing to do with your will power or lack thereof. Our bodies are being poisoned to the point of shut-down. Losing weight becomes fairly easy when we cut out chemicals, sugar, fillers, and processed carbohydrates. If you feel an increase in energy by the end of week one, it's a sure sign you were being affected by the sugars in your morning breakfast. Your body is at its most vulnerable in the morning, so it's easy to cause an all-day fog eating the wrong things in the morning. You might not even need as much coffee once this phase is complete and the sugars have been filtered out.

These first six weeks are going to be all about healing; you may not lose ANY weight during this time—none. Why? Because your body is literally turning back on and resetting, and this takes *time*... four to six weeks, in my experience. You may notice a change in your face almost immediately, however, and your pants may get a bit looser. This is because inflammation tends to fade immediately.

YOU CAN DO THIS! Your health is now up to you, but I promise I'll give you all of the tools you'll need to succeed.

WEEK 2

WEEK 2 CHALLENGE

This week we're getting the sugar out during the day, until dinnertime. This is going to be tough, but you can do it!

Week 2 has two parts: eating and moving. So, with no further ado:

Part One: Eating

Below are my favorite go-to lunches (see my sample diary for more suggestions). Focus on protein, and try to fill up on veggies, nuts, and berries. You can add yogurt too; you have lots of options.

- Salad piled high with meat, cheese, and veggies. We usually do a big chef salad two or three times a week—they're super filling and give you lots of good protein. Remember, lean meats are best but any meat is fine. Heck, throw some bacon in there if you want. It's okay! FAT IS GOOD FOR YOU! Make sure your dressing is low sugar without any crazy additives. Regular old ranch or Italian, things like that. Check your labels!

- Soup. Progresso Lite soups are quick and easy choices for lunch, especially when you throw some WASA crackers in there, or include some Laughing Cow cheese on crackers as a side.

- Mission brand low carb wraps can be used for a rollup sandwich, a quesadilla, or even a pizza—just throw on some tomato sauce, cheese, turkey, pepperoni, and BAM, you've got a healthy pizza! Delicious. Veggies are always great, whether as a side, on a pizza, or however you want to eat them.

Part Two: Movement.

I want you to start moving this week, three times for thirty minutes. I don't even care how you do it. Dance naked in your living room if you want. The only requirement is that you move non-stop for thirty minutes three times this week. Walking is a great option. Don't overwhelm yourself—slow and steady wins the race. This is a change for your whole life, so no need to go crazy. If you love to dance, then I highly suggest Dance Fitness with Jessica. She's got free routines on YouTube that are really fun, so check them out!

WEEK 2 HOMEWORK

You are going to start to documenting your changes this week.

Daily: weigh yourself each morning immediately after your first pee. Write down anything specific you notice about how you are feeling or looking.

Weekly (yes, each week): I want photos. Take some "before photos" from the front and side, and then just your face. These are great for encouragement when the scale isn't moving. Sometimes things are changing shape when your weight stays the same. I also want a waist measurement at the very least. If you want to do more measurements, fine, but I need to have waist measurement. I know this is a lot, but this is a big week and I know you can do it.

Go get 'em!

WEEK 2 ENCOURAGEMENT

This is an 8-week, slow-and-steady plan. I am not expecting any weight loss at this stage and neither should you. In fact, your weight may even go up! That's fine, don't worry! The first four weeks is focused on cleaning up what you eat, and the next four are all about adjusting those foods to get your body into the weight loss mode. I want your weight loss to be for your whole life, not just for a few weeks or months. I want you living and eating in an entirely new way. You didn't become unhealthy over night, and you won't become healthy overnight, so please, please, *PLEASE* give this time. You need your body and mind working together. It's scientific fact that the more quickly you lose weight the less likely you are to keep it off, so let's do this right! Don't freak out and sabotage yourself and the plan.

We'll get there!

WEEK 3

WEEK 3 CHALLENGE

This is a big week. I know this challenge is going to be tough, so it's the *only* thing I'm asking you to do this week.

Cut out *all* non-stevia-sweetened soda and sugary drinks. You don't need them and they're doing incalculable harm to your body. The good news is; I have a few fun beverages for you to try this week.

I know you can do this!

Just say no to junk!

Stick with no sugar until dinnertime—after dinner it is all yours…this week.

Stick with thirty minutes of movement three times a week.

Keep tracking your weight every day.

You've got this! Lots more to come. We've only just begun.

WEEK 3 ENCOURAGEMENT

Do you drink Green Tea? If not, you should! But drinking any tea will be great for you. Add some cinnamon and ginger to help with the detox and to keep your blood sugars level. I usually have some green tea about three in the afternoon, with a few nuts to keep me satisfied until dinner.

My afternoon tea treat, Wilder Tea:

- Steep your favorite green or black tea (make sure it doesn't have added gluten)
- Add some unsweetened vanilla almond milk
- Sprinkle on some cinnamon (this is going to help you fight sugar cravings)
- Add some ginger (so good for you! I buy it in both liquid and powder forms)
- Add a little Stevia if you are craving some sweetness.

Pro Tip: Don't forget to drink lots of water. Drinking water when you wake up in the morning will jump start your metabolism; add some lemon to get that fire burning!

WEEK 4

WEEK 4 CHALLENGE

This is a big one, so hold on to your Spanx!

This week we are cutting out ALL sugar and refined carbs. Kiss them all goodbye, because you don't need them—they're killing you! That's a bold statement, but it's the absolute truth. They're hurting you and you no longer want that, you want to be healthy and strong. This week you should see a pretty big difference in your face, so make sure to take a photo or two. All your inflammation is going to go away pretty quickly once we get all the junk out of your system. Get excited! Big things are about to happen.

The second part of the challenge this week is about movement. I'm not changing the three times a week movement rule, but I do want one of those days spent either walking, wogging, or jogging. Thirty minutes of your feet hitting the pavement. I don't care how fast or slow you go, just get out and do it. Even short bursts of wogging and getting your heart rate up is great for you. Try it!

You've got this!

WEEK 4 HOMEWORK REMINDER

Daily: I want you to weigh yourself each morning right after your first pee. I also want you to note anything specific about how you are feeling or looking.

Weekly: I want photos. Take some "before photos"; front and side views, and then also just your face. These are great for comparison and encouragement when the scale isn't moving. Sometimes things are changing shape when your weight stays the same. Remember to take your waist measurement. If you want to take more measurements, go right ahead, but make sure you do that waist measurement.

WEEK 4 ENCOURAGEMENT

Don't cry into your Wilder oats just yet! There are so many good things you can have this week! Low carb mission wraps, brown rice, sweet potatoes, sprouted breads, Dreamfields brand pasta, oats, quinoa, nut flours, and carbs that naturally occur in fruits, nuts, veggies and beans. You'll get the hang of this. It's okay for progress to take some time. It *will* happen and you *will* get there. Just stick with me and don't give up.

WEEK 5

WEEK 5 CHALLENGE
  BLACK PLATE WEEK

Remember, black plates are for proteins and fats; white plates are for proteins and carbs.

As I already said, our bodies have difficulty keeping our metabolism running steadily when we consume both high fats and high carbs in the same meal. So, this week and next week we are in fats and carbs boot camp. This week is the harder of the two, since it's BLACK PLATE WEEK. This means you won't be eating ANY carbs for the next week—your *only* bread choice is Mission brand low carb wraps.

No other grains.

AT ALL.

I'm watching you.

The only fruits allowed are berries, lemons and limes. Don't cry, though, because you can load up on cheese, sour cream, meats, nuts, and Lily's chocolate. Please be sure to take a look at my ***BLACK PLATE WEEK SHEET on page 287** for full food options.

KEEP MOVING

You also need to walk, run or wog for as long as you can this week. If possible, I want you to try my Wilder Wog, described in the FAQ section. Journal about it at home, and then let me know how it went. I want specifics like, "I walked for twenty minutes and I wogged for ten. It was really hard and I almost died and I hate you."

You can do this.

Be prepared to kick some serious ass.

Keep up on your daily weigh-ins and measurements! Change is a-comin'.

It's going to be worth it, I promise!

WEEK 5 ENCOURAGEMENT

My dream is to start a revolution, one in which we all stop dieting and begin a new regimen of eating that we will stick to for our whole lives. One where we start feeling good about our bodies, where we have positive self-images and we walk with our heads held high, proud of what we've accomplished. In this health and wellness revolution, everyone believes they can run—and they even get excited about it. I long for the day when we aren't suffering from horrible diseases like diabetes, PCOS and ADHD. I want the whole world to know that if *I* can do it, they can do it, too.

WEEK 6

WEEK 6 CHALLENGE
WHITE PLATE WEEK

Remember, black plates are for proteins and fats; white plates are for proteins and carbs.

This week is the same concept as last week, except we're changing plate colors; get out your white plates, girls, because this week the carbs are in the house!

Carbs have a bit of a bad reputation, but they aren't the bad nutrient everyone makes them out to be. You just need to find the *right* carbs to put on your plate—that's what we're doing this week, focusing on *healthy* carbs. Which means all other kinds of carbs are dead to you…FOREVER!

The stars of the show this week are sprouted breads and cereals, old-fashioned oats, fruit, brown rice, beans, and potatoes. These are the good carbs; please be sure to check my graphic on *white plates, on page 287, for the full list.

This week you need to stick to *lean* meats and proteins. What does that mean? Chicken and turkey breast, fish, venison, lean ground turkey and chicken (96% protein or higher), lean deli meats and ground beef—85% lean or better (drained). Make sure you stick to low fats in your food this week because we don't want to have any of our black plate friends accidentally turn your white plates gray—that is *not* allowed.

This week might seem hard, but I know you can do it. Just focus on lean protein and don't forget your veggies, as you'll need lots of fiber after the full week of fats last week.

Yes, you can still have Progresso light soup.

It will be okay, I promise!

You've got this!

WEEK 6 HOMEWORK:

Keep taking photos and measurements, and don't forget to journal. This is your health journey, so we want good records to show how far you've come!

This week we're also going to amp up your training. I need you to step it up…literally. Continue with the three movement sessions of at least thirty minutes each this week. Two of those *have* to be walking/wogging/jogging for as long as you can, as far as you can. I don't care what those numbers are, but you HAVE to try. You're going to be running a 5k soon, so we need to get you ready. Now get going! Get on your workout gear, ladies, because it's time to get moving!

WEEK 6 ENCOURAGEMENT

Are you starting to feel the changes in your body? Maybe your weight has gone down a bit, or maybe it's gone up. Regardless of the number, you're seeing and feeling *something*. This week and next week we're setting the metabolic pendulum into full swing. Think of your body as a beautiful beach: the black plate and white plate weeks will put the waves into motion. It's okay if you see your weight start to creep up a bit, that's normal. Just look for an overall, long-term downward trend. As we get into the next few weeks you'll see that now that your metabolism has been jump-started, keeping it revving will become easier and easier. Just keep on keeping on, have faith in your body and in the plan, and don't stop moving!

WEEK 7

WEEK 7 CHALLENGE
MIXING UP YOUR PLATES!

Remember, black plates are for proteins and fats; white plates are for proteins and carbs.

This is the week you've been waiting for! Now we start to mix up your plates. Throughout the last two weeks you've probably been able to see how your body responds differently to the protein plus fats combination, and the protein plus carbs combination. Now we're going to keep mixing it up so your body never knows what's coming.

An important note before we get started, though, is that you can't do this halfway. This *isn't* Atkins. Think about these two different plates like a swinging pendulum. As far as you swing in one direction, you need to swing just as far in the opposite direction. Don't be scared of good carbohydrates! Your body needs them. Swinging back and forth will keep the waves of your metabolism moving.

Try these daily plans this week and find out which one works best for you. Next week you'll be totally freestyling your plates, and even mixing them up a bit.

So, for Week 7, your job is to adhere to the following in terms of your food intake:

Day 1: Black only all day

Day 2: White only all day

Day 3: Black, Black, White—breakfast, lunch, dinner

Day 4: White, White, Black—breakfast, lunch, dinner

Day 5: Black, White, Black—breakfast, lunch, dinner

Day 6: White, Black, White—breakfast, lunch, dinner

Day 7: White, Black, Black—breakfast, lunch, dinner

As well, I want you wogging three times this week, for as long as you can. Stop and walk if you have to, but I want you to really push your limits this week.

Don't forget, your body was made for greatness!

WEEK 7 ENCOURAGEMENT:

Can you see the finish line? You're *so* close to reaching your goal! Your metabolism is running full force this week, you're wogging and starting to get strong. This is the time to journal. Remember how you're feeling, and don't forget it's only been less than two months. Can you believe how far you have come? Remember where you started, and keep an eye on where you're going! That 5k will be here before you know it!

WEEK 8

WEEK 8 CHALLENGE
PLATES YOUR WAY!

Remember, black plates are for proteins and fats; white plates are for proteins and carbs.

Eating:

Congratulations! You made it to Week 8! Four weeks of detox, three weeks of learning plate styles and combinations, and now this final week where we get your metabolism revving high and on fire—not just for a few weeks or months, but for the rest of your life!

This week is all about learning how to keep it going on your own.

All you need to do is pick your plate for each meal; ask yourself which plate do you want for this meal? Which color will you do for breakfast tomorrow, or dinner on Thursday? This is the easy part, really, because you are totally in control. You can mix it up however you want!

A word of caution, though: don't devise your meal plan to include fifty plates of gray! Gray plates are, of course, plates that combine carbs, fats, and proteins. You don't want too many gray plates in your weekly plan—I try to limit mine to about three or four per week, max. Gray plates are totally fine in moderation, and they will help keep you on the right path, just don't get too dependent on them. We need to keep that pendulum always moving, those waves always crashing.

Now that we have your body working *for* you rather than against you, you have to keep working for your body. How many black plates and how many white plates should you do per week? Well, that depends on you; your body will tell you what it needs. I try to get in one white plate each day, usually for breakfast, as I've found this the best way to keep my metabolism humming at a nice pace. You may find yourself needing more white plates or fewer, depending on how your body responds.

I do think, however, that the more you increase physical activity the more white plates you'll probably need, since they're a great energy source. If you're doing a long or strenuous run, I would make sure you have a white plate dinner the night before and then again for breakfast that morning—you'll need those carbs! I do average more black plates than white, and more white than gray, but that's just what works best for me as a borderline diabetic. Everyone is different; so let your body dictate what's best for you.

If you stall in terms of weight loss, my best advice is to mix things up. Keep changing up the plate colors and that'll get things moving. Don't worry when you have those stalls, though—your body just needs time to adjust. I hit a plateau about every fifteen to twenty pounds I lose.

Don't forget to hydrate.

Eat your veggies.

EAT! Not eating enough, regardless of plate color, will only slow your progress. Try to get to a place where you're neither under-eating nor over-eating, and don't forget that protein is *always* the focus.

These basic principles will keep your body moving and healthy.

Movement:

Your movement this week is easy: Three days of wogging, working up to a 5k!

- Day 1: one easy mile. Walk first and then try to move into a wog and keep wogging as much as you can.
- Day 2: two miles. Start with a nice brisk walk and work into your wog. Wog to the end. Don't forget to "beast mode" those last few minutes!
- Day 3: three miles! Yes, *three*. You can totally just walk the first one, nice and easy. Mile two, get into a comfortable wogging pace. Bring it back down to a walk whenever you need. Mile three is for beast mode: push yourself hard! Find out how much wogging you can do all the way to the finish line. You've totally got this 5k in the bag!

I knew you could do it, even when you didn't!

Now, just keep it up on your own.

Keep training and keep moving your body.

You're kicking ass!

WEEK 8 HOMEWORK:

Keep documenting your changes.

Daily: Keep weighing yourself each morning right after your first pee. I also want you to note anything specific you noticed about how you're feeling or looking.

Weekly: I want photos. Take some "before photos"; front and side, and then also just your face. Use these photos for comparison purposes when the scale isn't moving. Sometimes things are changing shape when your weight stays the same. Keep up with those waist measurements and if you want to do more measurements, fine, but don't stop putting that measuring tape around your waist. I would love to hear your story and see your photos! Please consider emailing them to me, or sharing on social media. www.jasindawilder.com **#biggirlsdoitrunning**

WEEK 8 ENCOURAGEMENT:

Give your body as long as it takes to reach a place of strength and health. How long will that be? Eight more weeks? Eight more months? Eighteen months? It doesn't matter! The only goal is good health. If there's anything I've learned on this journey, it's to give my body time and grace: this isn't a sprint, it's a marathon. Don't worry if you trip up a few times along the way—just pick yourself up and keep on wogging. You've made all the right steps toward good health, now keep focused on the next meal, the next day, and the next run.

I'm so proud of you!

Pro tip: I tend to "Suzan Sommersize" my fruit, meaning eating it in moderation and eating it alone, unless it's berries, lemons, or limes. I've found loading fruit in with other carbs is just too much sugar for me, and I suspect you may find the same thing to be true for you.

PART 5

Additional Info to Keep You Motivated

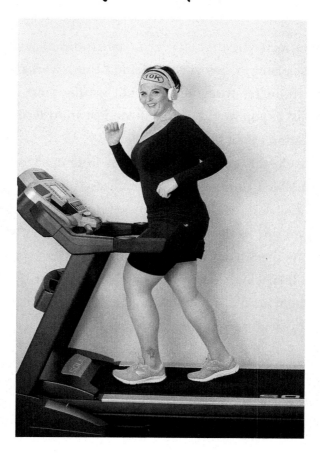

Jasinda's Reset:

FOR THOSE TIMES WHEN YOU JUST NEED A KICK-START.

I F YOU FEEL AS IF YOU JUST CAN'T GET THE HANG OF WHICH ORDER to do your plates in, below is a version I think works well for the long term. If you're struggling with not getting your metabolism moving as fast as you would like, or if you just aren't feeling so great, this combination might be helpful to you.

I like to do this combination with as little dairy on my black plates as possible—think a sprinkle of cheese instead of a full cup. You can still have it, just cut back on your cheese, cream, and any other dairy for one week and see how you feel. I also try to limit myself to just one snack a day when I'm doing this little reset. If I get the munchies, I'll snack on some non-starchy veggies or berries. Keep your movement normal and don't forget to drink lots of water; I like to infuse mine with some lemon and lime.

- Day 1: B-B-B
- Day 2: B-W-B
- Day 3: B-W-B
- Day 4: W-B-B
- Day 5: B-W-B
- Day 6: W-B-B

- Day 7: B-B-W

You can come back to this whenever you need a week of reset. Sometimes we can get too much dairy, which can block us up or slow us down, and I think this is a nice little break for our body. I know mine really likes it.

FAQS

What happens if I mess up? Why will it be different this time?

"I can't do this."

"I messed up."

"I'm a failure."

"I ate a cupcake."

"I didn't run this week."

"This can't work for me."

"I'm hopeless."

I've said all those things to myself at some point on this journey. Here's the reality.

So what if you ate something you shouldn't have? So what if you skipped a whole week of working out! So what if you're sure when you step on the scale tomorrow you'll have gained twenty pounds? This kind of thinking is something we need to toss out the window, *permanently*.

Let me fill you in on a little secret: you aren't perfect. Why are you expecting yourself to be? You *are* going to mess up. Everyone does, at some point. You might have a bad day, or even a bad week, but that doesn't mean you give up! Dust yourself off and try again. Don't even dwell on the failure, because that isn't going to help anyone, least of all you. When's your next meal? Focus on that! Do that one right. This is a day-by-day, meal-by-meal plan. Ignore minor slip-ups; focus instead on all the amazing things you're accomplishing, focus on everything you're doing right.

You're going to finish a 5k! You're going to work your body and get stronger and healthier. This isn't a "maybe", this is fact. Pay no attention to unimportant hiccups and focus on your future. Remember why you are doing this. Think about the people you are going to inspire. It's okay to mess up every so often, just keep your eyes on the prize.

Food combinations and carb cycling: Why does it work?

When I was pregnant with my daughter I had a come-to-Jesus revelation. As I explained earlier, my body was literally prego-craving food combinations. I would eat eggs and bacon for breakfast, a big chef salad for lunch, and maybe some whole grains at dinner. I never ate fats and carbs together because it literally made me feel ill. I have no explanation for this phenomenon. I had huge bursts of energy, which was also odd because I was pregnant. And perhaps most important, I didn't want sugar *at all*—even the thought of sugar nauseated me. I started wondering what was going on with me. I didn't realize it at the time, but I was food combining and it was making me feel good.

I searched Google for recipes that were low-carb and no-sugar, and I kept hitting on Trim Healthy Mama recipes. Do yourself a HUGE favor and get that cookbook, it's amazing. They talk about food combining and cycling, too. And then I read several more books that each confirmed what I was starting to believe: eating fats and carbohydrates in the same meal makes it difficult to lose weight—in fact, I believe eating those two things together frequently makes it nearly impossible. The problem is with the fact that we've created foods that are impossible to digest. The result is that many of us have slow, lagging, messed up metabolisms. By eating foods that are over processed and full of unnatural, inedible chemicals we've clogged up our systems. Giving your body similar natural foods in logical groupings will turn on your metabolic engine.

I don't believe in taking away an entire food group—like a carb-free diet for example. I just don't think it's sustainable or smart. But I *do* believe in jumpstarting your metabolism with food combinations that will make it dramatically easier to lose weight. Along with making some other adjustments and changes in your life, food combining will help you win the impossible weight loss struggle you've fought against your whole life.

It's a light bulb moment.

Yes, you can eat pasta, rice, and the occasional potato. You can have meat. You can have cake and ice cream—as long as it's made with stevia. I don't want you to be deprived; I want you to be healthy and smart. If you don't believe me, read some of the books written on the subject by actual doctors, who know much more than I do and can explain it more thoroughly. There is a list of these books at the end of this book.

Or, you can give me eight weeks and see what happens.

What results can I expect if I follow your 8-Week Plan?

Here's what will happen if you follow my program:

- Normal, stable blood sugar levels
- Increased energy
- Better complexion

- Better sleep patterns
- Increased strength (both mental and physical)
- Better focus
- Reduced inflammation
- Weight loss
- Self confidence

I know these are bold statements to make.

I know I might even sound crazy.

I've tested my plan with objective groups of women who were as frustrated as I was with continuing to fail at successfully completing weight loss plans. I also recruited friends, my family, my children and my husband, not to mention myself. Every single person who tried my method experienced the benefits listed above.

Why is my plan different?

Because it works.

Because combining the body and mind is just as important as combining foods.

Just try it for 8 weeks—don't rush and don't skip any steps. You won't figure this all out overnight. Give your body the grace and time it needs. You're in this for life. I'll be here with you!

Why the different plate colors?

It's the best way I've found to make the plan easy to understand.

It's simple: black plates are for proteins and fats; white plates are for proteins and carbs. Gray plates contain carbs, fats, and proteins, but use them in moderation.

And no, you don't need to go out and buy all new dishes and only use black, white, or gray plates. I simply devised this as an easy way to visualize the different meal options and combinations.

Why aren't there any fat or carb limits on these plates?

Because only you know your body, and I believe in listening to what your body is telling you, and eating until you are full. Your build, gender, age, and exercise level can also affect the amount your body may need, so setting generalized limits doesn't work; just don't over eat. You don't need to eat everything on your plate; enjoy your food, eat until you're full, and try to keep your body guessing. Which plate is coming next? Only you know; there are no rules.

What do I eat when I'm at a restaurant?

Don't worry! We eat out all the time, so I've got you covered. You can eat almost anywhere and find something that will leave you feeling satisfied and proud of yourself for not eating something harmful to your body. I can even find something at the bar to eat! Imagine it, a mother of six hanging out at the bar and sticking to her health plan.

Below is a quick list of ideas to help you be successful wherever you dine:

- Focus on protein—just about every restaurant is going to have meat. What's your favorite? Beef, chicken, seafood? Figure out a way to have it prepared the way you want it. Talk to the server and explain your needs. Most chefs are hip to the needs of their customers, and most of them have no trouble adjusting a dish to suit you. If a Starbuck's barista can pull off a Grande, Quad, Nonfat, One-Pump, No-Whip, Mocha then I'm pretty sure a chef can wrangle a no-carb or a no-sugar meal.

- Even at a drive thru or a deli counter, don't be afraid to ask for things to be prepared the way you want them; you're paying for this food and you should be able to order it the way you like it. Don't be embarrassed to ask for a lettuce wrap for your burger instead of a bun. It's okay; you aren't the only one doing it! We have two restaurants in our town that are now doing a burger lettuce wrap option because of us! Start a trend, be cool!

- Start with a side salad
- Forget the chips and salsa, and order some veggies and guacamole instead
- Grilled fajitas without the tortillas
- Taco or grilled chicken salad—just pick a dressing that isn't too sweet; creamy is best, or just oil and vinegar
- Tacos in a lettuce wrap, or just eat the filling.
- A burrito in a bowl without the wrap
- A big bowl of chili
- Omelets with bacon or sausage
- Plain chicken wings—always ask for sauce on the side, as you don't need as much as you think
- Grilled salmon with brown rice—always ask if it's really brown or just white rice colored to look brown, or choose a sweet potato instead of the rice
- Lettuce wrap or unwich—ask your favorite burger joint or deli to wrap with lettuce: most will gladly do this for you.
- At a pizza place? Go for the wings, or get a salad and throw the entire pizza toppings, cheese and all, on top. You won't believe how yummy that is!

Pro tip: You don't need bread, and you don't need croutons, but if you are anything like me you NEED some wine. That's okay! Just pick something red and dry. Don't like it dry? Throw some stevia in it when the waiter isn't looking—he'll never know. Don't like wine? Have a low carb beer or two. Vodka and La Croix is also a great choice, and whiskey is Mr. Wilder's favorite.

Isn't it more expensive eating this way?

Yes and no. Yes, your food bill might go up a tiny bit, but not as much as you might expect. When you aren't buying all the highly marketed, packaged junk, you'll find your family is eating a smaller quantity of the nutrient-packed good stuff, which means the kids won't be asking for snacks every thirty minutes. You'll stay full longer and you'll have more energy so you won't need the quick fix from sugar and carbohydrates.

I did see a slight increase in our food bill during the first few weeks because we did a lot of stocking up on new ingredients. Once we had completely changed over into the healthier eating pattern, we didn't see much change in our grocery bill.

Shopping is actually *much* easier because I know all the items we eat and I just load up on those when I see a good price on them. There aren't any impulse buys, and I'm no longer tempted by slick marketing and packaging—even my kids can see right through that crap, now. The other huge money savings comes from better health: being sick is expensive! My family is so much healthier since we've started eating this way, and our overall quality of life is just better. We eat better food, feel better, and live better.

So even if there is a small monetary increase, I believe it is well worth it. I'd rather invest in my health than anything else.

Why does my weight keep going up and down?

I wish I had a really smart and savvy scientific answer for that. The truth is I can only link the weight fluctuations to water weight and your monthly cycle. So, to me, this is very, very normal. My best suggestion is to keep close track of your weight; I highly recommend using an app that will show you the overall downward trend of your loss. I like the Happy Scale app for that because it clearly shows that even if you go up by a few pounds this week or that, your overall weight loss is still trending down.

I really wish I'd had a better grasp on all of this when I first started my new plan—I'd gain five pounds in the middle of the month, every single month, and it drove me *crazy*. Once I really started paying attention and tracking it, however, I found out it was just water weight associated with ovulation. I know some people will tell you not to weigh yourself every single day, but I believe the scale is simply a tool we can use to better understand our bodies. It's important to keep in mind the number on the scale is just that, a number, but what those numbers can tell us may actually help us feel better.

Everyone is different. I now know that each month my weight loss is part of a cycle I can predict: week one, I'll go down maybe a pound or two; week two, my weight usually goes up; week three, I'm down four pounds; week four, I'm going to lose a few more pounds. This is a consistent cycle for me. On average I lose about a pound or two a week. If I was on week two and I saw that gain I might even give up—don't do it! Weight fluctuations like that are absolutely normal, so don't freak out. We're looking for a downward trend over the *long* term.

Just keep doing what you're doing. You're making great progress! This is NOT a quick loss program; this is slow and steady, these are healthy changes for the rest of your life. One pound a week is great! That's fifty-two pounds a year! Don't get caught up in the numbers; get caught up in taking control over your health and how you feel. Don't let anything steal the joy of your success.

You're doing great!

What is Wilder Wogging, and how do I do it?

Wogging is my low impact version of running—I would almost

call it a shuffle. I try to land flat on the middle of my feet to make sure that my whole foot is taking the impact rather than just my heel. My feet stay low to the ground and I make sure to tighten my stomach and butt as much as possible, which has the added benefit of really helping to tighten and strengthen those areas.

You can wog as fast or as slow as you want, just take it one step at a time and gradually increase your speed. If you do have bad knees, please remember to reduce the impact by keeping your feet low to the ground—meaning, don't lift your knees or feet too much, which is why it feels more like a fast shuffle than anything else. You might feel a bit like you're falling forward, but that assist from gravity will actually make it easier for you to keep going.

Don't worry if you need to slow to a walk for a minute and then pick it back up; my kids can actually walk faster than I wog, and that's just fine. The wog part just adds to the cardio aspect and helps my momentum. Check out YouTube for a video about how to wog, or find me online if you need more help!

Happy wogging!

What happens when I reach all my goals?

First, congratulations! Next, I would challenge you to set new goals! If you feel happy with the weight you're at, great! Do you feel physically fit and strong? Awesome! If you're getting to the point that you're worried about losing *too* much I'd start adding in more whole grains and good carbohydrates with your high fat meals. It's okay! My husband and children always do a side of brown rice, whole grain bread, whole grain pasta or a potato to maintain their size and energy. Once you feel like you're in a good place, those carbs will help maintain your weight—just don't add in added sugars, those will *always* get you in trouble.

What do I do with all this skin?

That is an excellent question! If you figure it out, let me know! My best advice is to get a good pair of Spanx; those things work wonders. I have tried a few other things like skin brushing and cellulite lotions, but none of them did much for me. I think if you lose a significant amount of weight, skin is just going to be an issue for you unless you're blessed with some miracle genetics.

There are surgical options for skin removal, but those also come with risks. I can't say I haven't thought about having surgery, because the excess skin on my thighs rubs a lot and I do find it really makes running more difficult. At this point, though, I'm not sure I'm willing to undergo another surgery. In the end, I think you need to do what makes *you* feel good. You've come a long way, and you deserve to feel as good as you can in your skin.

Have you only tested this plan on your family?

No, I would never publish a book like this without doing objective testing to make sure my plan can help a wide variety of people. A beta test group worked with me over the course of several months helping me to tweak my health plan. These ladies did a phenomenal job with my program, so please be sure to read their testimonials at the end of the book.

My testers came from different backgrounds and ages, and they all had different reasons for wanting to change their health. They all saw positive results from the changes they made on my program. One of my beta group ladies hadn't seen a normal blood sugar reading since she was thirteen, but after only three weeks on my program she was seeing normal numbers. Another found relief from issues with her period, and another saw better overall energy with her struggles with MS. Most of these ladies also included their children in the new healthy eating plan and they saw great results, too.

I'm positive my health plan will bring about positive results for anyone who does the full eight weeks as I've laid them out. Cutting out added sugar and refined carbohydrates along with eating healthy and whole foods will do wonders for everyone.

Why is it okay for me to eat fruit and dairy?

Well, maybe it is and maybe it isn't—I think that's something you need to really watch and figure out while doing my 8-week plan. Are you sensitive to dairy? If so, limit how much you have, or cut it from your diet entirely. If something makes you feel bloated, gassy, or in pain, then stop eating it! I think for most of us a moderate amount of cheese, sour cream, or yogurt is going to be okay. Just pay attention to your own body and make adjustments if you feel better without a certain type of food.

Fruit is the same. Personally, I can't eat too much fruit; I *love* my berries, but a banana will make me feel yucky if I have it with too many other healthy carbs. I know that several people in my BETA group were able to enjoy apples, bananas, and even other fruits with no issue at all. If you have pre-diabetes or diabetes, then I would caution you to really watch the fructose. A steady insulin level will ensure the best health for you. Moderation and self-evaluation is key here.

Should I add other forms of exercise?

I think walking/wogging and jogging are the best exercises to start out with. I would try my gradual approach with the eight-week plan and then see how you feel. You could add a few other forms of cardio; jump rope is a killer workout, and I love to challenge my sons with it. Aerobic dancing is also really fun—my daughter and I to do it together. You could do some kettlebells or light weights for strength training if you feel like it. I don't think strength workouts will contribute to weight loss, but it's all about how you feel. Listen to your body and add things when you are ready. This is a marathon, not a sprint. Take your time and find your own health groove.

How do I make peace with my body?

Focus on all the good things it's done for you. It's time to love yourself and your body. You've come such a long way! Be proud of yourself and all the things you've done with your body so far. Comparison is the thief of joy. This is your journey, your race. Take it one day at a time, one meal at a time, and one wog at a time. You'll get there!

DAILY MEAL SUGGESTIONS

Keep it simple! One day at a time, one meal at a time.

Day 1: (Black, Black, Black)

Breakfast: Cheese and salsa omelets with a side of bacon or sausage.

Lunch: Chef salad with no-sugar-added dressing.

Dinner: Cheeseburger without a bun and a side of broccoli and/or green beans.

Snacks: Almonds or WASA crackers with laughing cow cheese, Oikos Triple Zero Yogurt

Day 2: (White, White, Black)

Breakfast: Old Fashioned Oats with unsweetened almond milk and Greek yogurt and berries. (Wilder morning mush—see recipe)

Lunch: Quesadilla with a Mission low-carb wrap, lean meat, peppers and Laughing Cow cheese . A few blue corn chips and fresh salsa

Dinner: Burger or Salmon over salad. (If your kids don't like salmon you can also use plain chicken strips. My kids love to make their own bowls, so don't toss your salad; let them pick what they want for toppings. You'll be surprised what they might pick. I often do some berries as a side, and maybe some rice, too.)

Snacks: protein shake (I love Jay Robb with some Greek yogurt, stevia, integral collagen, and berries—see recipe); almonds and cheese

Day 3: (Black, White, Black)

Breakfast: Breakfast burrito on Mission low carb wrap. Eggs, bacon or sausage, cheese, peppers or onions, or just some *pico de gallo*.

Lunch: Light soup (we love Progresso Lite) and some WASA crackers, and a Triple Zero yogurt

Dinner: Spaghetti with Dreamfield's pasta. I use spaghetti sauce made with ground turkey but with no added sugar, and we top it with cheese. We include a side of vegetables. Let your kids pick which ones they want. Also add a side salad and eat that first.

Snacks: Berries, Quest bar, some Lily's chocolate

Day 4: (Black, Black, Black)

Breakfast: Cheese omelet seasoned with sea salt and some cayenne pepper. Side of Applegate chicken sausage.

Lunch: Large Chef Salad

Dinner: Wilder Wings, salad, and veggies

Snacks: Quest Bar, almonds and cashews

Day 5: (White, White, Black)

Breakfast: Protein loaded pancakes (see recipe). You can leave out the chocolate chips.

Lunch: Mission wrap sandwiches with lean meat and Laughing Cow cheese

Dinner: Homemade pizza using Mission low carb wraps (Fat Head low carb crust is another great option)

Snack: sugar free Cheesecake (see recipe)

Day 6: (White, Black, White)

Breakfast: Scrambled egg whites and toast

Lunch: Chili (see recipe)

Dinner: Loaded sweet potato and/or grilled chicken kabobs

Snack: nuts, Nanny Karri cookies

Day 7: (White, Black, Black)

Breakfast: Triple Zero yogurt, berries and toast (mix some Ezekiel almond or flax cereal into the yogurt for extra fiber)

Lunch: Lettuce wrapped burger (so yummy!)

Dinner: Pizza cups (see recipe)

Snack: Quest bar

Pro Tip: White plates are MADE for wogging. If you're going t(be doing a big run or workout, a white plate meal is a great ide because it's fast burning. I love having oatmeal or pancakes ma with oats for some extra pep in my step.

SAMPLE RUNNING DIARY

Day 1: Today I didn't really want to run but I got out there and ran a whole mile. I only stopped twice. My pace was 17 minutes per mile and I felt pretty good when I was done. Go me!

After run snack: Quest bar

Day 2: Today I ran a bit further than yesterday, but I stopped three times. One time I actually thought I might die. The middle of my run felt best. Tomorrow I'm going to rest.

After run snack: protein shake

Day 3: Rest Day. (Yes, Rest days and weeks are important—your body needs the rest to rebuild those muscles)

Day 4: Didn't have time to run.

Day 5: I RAN TWO MILES! Not full-out running, but not as slow as a walk. I felt great when I was finished. I only stopped once.

After run snack: Triple Zero yogurt

Day 6: Rest Day
Day 7: I took the dog and kids for a nice 30-minute walk. I told the kids I wanted to see them run and we wogged for about half of it. It was so much fun to exercise with them! I'm feeling better and stronger every day!

Snack: Mixed berries topped with Fat Free Reddi whip (one of my very favorite snacks).

Pro Tip: *It doesn't matter if you run or walk outside or inside. All that matters is that you did it. Figure out how you like to move and get moving!*

Jasinda's Jams

WORK MY BODY WORKOUT PLAYLIST

I LOVE TO LISTEN TO MUSIC AS I WALK, WOG, OR JOG. BELOW ARE some great tunes that get me motivated and moving.

"Levels"—Avicii

"Till the World Ends"—Britney Spears

"Chasing the Sun"—The Wanted (Hardwell Radio Edit)

"Don't Wake Me Up"—Chris Brown (Panic City Remix)

"Stronger" —Kelly Clarkson (Nicky Romero Club Mix)

"The One That Got Away"—Katy Perry (R3had club mix)

"Hey Mama"—David Guetta (Club Killers Remix)

"G.D.F.R." —Flo Rida (Nolaswift Remix)

"Time of Our Lives"—Ne-Yo & Pitbull (DJ Noodles Remix)

"Where Are U Now"—Skrillex and Diplo with Justin Bieber (Kaskade Remix)

"Outside"—Calvin Harris feat. Ellie Goulding (Hardwell Remix)

"Shut Up and Dance"—Walk The Moon (Jason Nevins Remix) *

"Something Better" —Audien (feat. Lady Antebellum) *

"Love Myself"—Hailee Steinfeld *

"Turn Down For What"—DJ Snake & Lil John

"Work"—Iggy Azalea (Gregor Salto Radio Edit)

"Fireball"—Pitbull feat. John Ryan (Jump Smokers Remix)

"Stay With Me"—Sam Smith (Soul Clap Remix)

"Work Work"—Britney Spears *

"Lose Yourself"—Eminem

"Black Horse"—Katy Perry

"Burn"—Ellie Goulding (Mat Zo Remix)

"Neon Lights"—Demi Levato (Country Club Martini Remix)

"I Cry"—Flo Rida *

"Must Be Love"—Christina Grimmie *

"WTF (Where They From)" —Missy Elliott

"Light It Up"—Major Lazer (feat. Nyla & Fuse ODG)

"Work This Body"—Walk The Moon

"Drop It Low"—Kat DeLuna

*ONE OF JASINDA'S FAVORITES – A MUST HAVE!

Pro Tip: The Spotify and Rock My Run apps will use your smart phone to monitor your running pace and suggest music to match your pace. Rock My Run has really improved my run time. It's also a great way to find new running music that will keep in rhythm with your own movement.

BUSY MOM AND WILDER KID APPROVED RECIPES

MY KIDS ARE ALWAYS GIVEN THE OPTION OF A HEALTHY CARB as a side with dinner. They're growing so they need those good, healthy carbs for energy! I know you're busy too, so you don't need a bunch of fancy recipes to keep your family healthy and happy, you just need a few dozen tried-and-true recipes your whole family will love. Figure out what they like and modify them to be healthy. It'll be easier than you think, trust me on this. You're laying the health groundwork for your child's entire life—making these changes now will improve their health forever.

For full-color recipe photos, please visit www.biggirlsdoitrunning. com.

Wild(er) Monkey cakes
(White/Gray Plate)

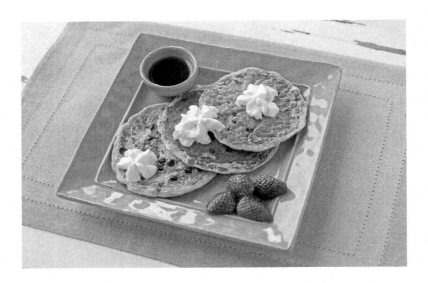

These are our Saturday or Sunday morning go-to special treat for our kids. I won't even tell you how long it takes to make pancakes for eight people, but it's worth it to see the smiles on their faces. My kids look forward to waking up on the weekends now, because they smell breakfast and come running. We pair these with some turkey bacon.

Ingredients:

2 cups of oats, blend well in a blender or food processor and set aside

Blend together separately:

1 cup low fat cottage cheese

1 5.3oz container of Triple Zero yogurt (banana)

2 cups liquid egg whites (one large carton)

1 teaspoon vanilla extract

1 teaspoon banana extract

4 teaspoons baking powder

4 tablespoons stevia sweetener (Pyure or Swerve)

(You can also add a scoop of protein powder for added protein and a thicker texture).

Coconut oil (to grease the pan)

Method:

Blend all ingredients together, including the oats, and then let it sit for a while to thicken up. This is an important step, so don't skip it!

Heat your griddle or pan and lightly coat the surface with some coconut oil and cook on low heat.

I make these in four small frying pans. They are a bit thin—something between a crepe and a regular pancake.

Added notes:

Feel free to adjust the extract and yogurt flavors.

For the kids top the pancakes with fat free Redi whip, and/or sprinkle them with Lily's chocolate chips.

Keep them white plate for the adults.

Make sure you coat the pan with coconut oil, and cook on low heat.

Wild(er) Nachos
(These can be modified for any plate color)

My family LOVES nachos. My recipe is a worry-free way to enjoy an old favorite—I use sliced peppers instead of tortilla chips. Adjust the quantities to suit your needs.

Ingredients:
Bell peppers sliced into nacho-chip sized strips.

Sautéed ground beef, pork, turkey, or chicken. The seasoning is up to you.

Shredded cheddar cheese

Lettuce, hot peppers, salsa, onions, sour cream, green onions, tomatoes. Your choice.

Method:
Pre-heat the oven to 350 F

Place the peppers in an ovenproof baking dish

Place the cooked meat on top of the peppers

Sprinkle everything with the shredded cheese

Bake at 350 F for 5–10 minutes, or until the cheese is melted

Top with the lettuce, hot peppers, salsa, sour cream etc.

Option:
Make a cheese sauce by combining:

- 8oz grated sharp cheddar cheese
- 8th tsp cayenne pepper
- salt ¼ tsp
- ½ cup almond milk
- ½ cup cream cheese

- 1 tablespoon butter

Pour over the nachos and enjoy!

You can do these so many different ways. If I'm really in a hurry I'll throw the sliced peppers in the oven with just seasoning, salsa, and cheese. You can top them with so many fun things. Get creative!

Nanny Karri Cookies
(Black Plate)

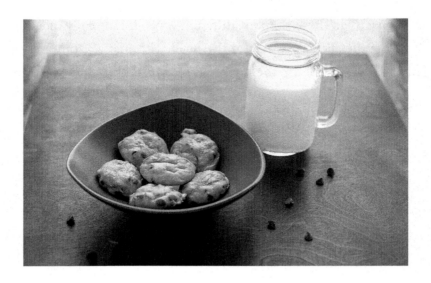

I found this recipe online and our nanny was super bummed because she couldn't eat them—she's allergic to almonds, the poor thing! She tried modifying the recipe so she could enjoy them, and ta-dah... Nanny Karri cookies! These cookies are soft and tasty and totally hit the cookie spot; you won't even miss your old sugar-filled cookies anymore. I promise!

"These cookies are so good, it makes me angry"- Jack Wilder

Ingredients:
8 oz 1/3 fat cream cheese (softened)
2 Tbsp butter
1 Tbsp natural peanut butter
1 cup stevia or stevia blend
1 tsp vanilla extract

Method:

Pre-heat the oven to 350 F

Line a cookie sheet with parchment paper

Whip everything in the above list until well combined

Then add:

Add 3 eggs

Keep whipping until the eggs are well combined

Then add:

½ tsp sea salt

½ tsp xantham gum (can be found online); it makes the cookies thick and chewy

1 tsp baking powder

2/3 cup peanut flour

1 scoopful whey protein powder (we use either vanilla or peanut butter—Jay Robb and Quest are my two favorite brands)

1½ cups Lily's brand sugar-free chocolate chips (you could also use the 70% dark cocoa variety)

Chopped nuts (these are optional)

Place spoonfulls of the batter on the cookie sheet

Bake at 350 degrees for 10 minutes.

This recipe makes about 50 cookies, but don't eat them all at once!

Wilder Mush
(white plate)

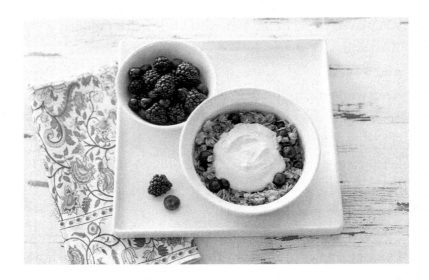

My kids *loved* the sugary, pre-packaged oatmeal—the kind with the dinosaur eggs that melt into dinosaur shaped sugar flakes was their favorite. I know, I know...*so* bad for them! Which meant, of course, that I had to find something to replace those little sugar bags of death. When I first started playing around with this recipe, I would add a few pinches of stevia to it in order for them to really like it, but now they don't miss the sweetener at all. Even if you aren't a kid—even if you don't really like oatmeal—give this a try. I've already converted most of my northern Michigan friends to this—it's perfect for those cold winter mornings. It'll hit the spot and keep you full till lunch.

For a single serving:

Ingredients:
1 to 1 ½ or 2 cups of old fashioned oats (you decide how hungry you are); Jack always needs two cups

Unsweetened vanilla almond milk

Frozen berries

Okios Triple Zero yogurt (single serving size)

Method:

Place the oats in a bowl and pour over the almond milk until it covers the oats (you don't want too much or it will taste watery—yuck)

Microwave on high for 2 or 2 ½ minutes

Top with some frozen berries and microwave for another 30 seconds.

Remove from microwave and mix in the container of Oikos Triple Zero yogurt.

Enjoy!

Note: Mix up the yogurt flavors and change the berries for different flavor combinations. We like the blueberry, raspberry, strawberry, blackberry and cherry flavors. Our favorite combos are raspberry vanilla and blueberry banana.

Jack and Jasinda's Chef's Salad
(Black Plate)

Jack and I eat a chef's salad almost every day; there are some days when we might have a tin of Progresso soup, or a rollup, but most days we do a salad. Jack usually has some WASA crackers with his, and I'll add some almonds or cashews as my side.

Ingredients:
A mixture of greens
Sliced meats: ham, turkey, chicken—whatever you like
Hard-boiled egg
Avocado
Tomatoes
Onions
Cheese
Salad Dressing of your choice

Method:
Layer everything into a pretty bowl and top with the dressing.

Notes:
We use a super-food greens mix available from our farmer's co-op that's got everything in it *except* iceberg lettuce. Branch out and try all the great greens that are out there like spinach or kale. Just try adding a bit more variety in terms of greens to your normal salad… you'll like it. Also, they have *way* more nutrients than iceberg lettuce.

Sometimes we'll add cheese crisps instead of regular cheese. Cheese crisps are made from baked cheese—sorta like a crouton without all the nasty crap. Yum! You can find them at your grocery store, probably in the produce section.

Right now we're really into the yogurt or salsa ranch dressings.

Some days I add a few squirts of lemon flavor fish oil when Jack isn't looking. Please don't tell him!

If you wanted to get really crazy, you could fold your salad inside a Mission Low Carb whole-wheat wrap.

It's such a quick and easy lunch—there's not a ton of prep and it fills us up for a long time. We're even lucky enough to have a local deli that knows our salad preferences, and they start making those salads for us as soon as we walk in!

Wilder Wings
(Black plate)

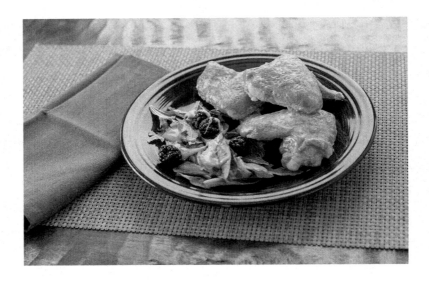

My kids *love* chicken wings! We usually go to Buffalo Wild Wings after church on Sunday because KIDS EAT HALF OFF! Do you know what a deal that is for parents with six kids? It's basically like winning the chicken wing lottery.

Well, my crazy kids kept hounding me to make my own wings, so I said, "Fine, I'll try." These are what I came up with. My family tends to like things a bit spicy, with lots of flavor, but you can adjust the spiciness to satisfy your little wild ones.

Ingredients:
40-50 chicken pieces: wings, thighs or strips. (For the health benefits, I prefer chicken on the bone, but little ones might prefer the strips).

6 tbsp Baking Powder

4 tsp salt

Method:

Preheat oven to 250 degrees

Wash and dry the chicken and place on a baking sheet lined with aluminum foil

Combine the baking powder and salt and then sprinkle over the chicken

Place the chicken on the middle or lower rack and cook for 30 minutes.

Then, while the chicken bakes, mix together in a small dish:

1 cup mayo

1 big spoonful of Greek yogurt

1 tbsp lime juice (bottled is fine)

½ cup to 1 cup (depending on spiciness preference) Frank's Red Hot Original Cayenne Pepper Sauce

½ tsp onion powder

½ tsp chili powder

½ tsp turmeric

A generous dash of Worchester sauce

½ tsp minced garlic

1 tbsp blackstrap molasses

pinch of pepper

Remove the chicken from the oven and turn up the oven temperature to 400 degrees.

Brush the chicken generously with the above mix. Bake for another 30 minutes at 400 degrees.

Pass the napkins!

Mere's Mixed Berry Muffins
(White plate)

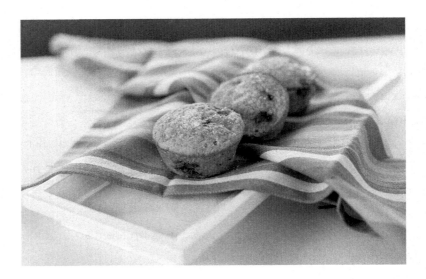

Meredith started helping me at home when we first moved up north and were further away from our parents; she's a real life Mary Poppins! She helps with everything from booking my hotel rooms to picking up kids from school, so when we started making our big health changes, she helped me by grabbing things at the grocery store and preparing meals. She's amazing, and so are her muffins!

These muffins freeze well and they are great to have on hand when you're having a hectic morning.

Ingredients:
1 cup oat flour
½ cup coconut flour
3 tsp baking powder
1 cup Swerve
6 tbsp water

1¾ cup egg whites

¼ tsp sea salt

¾ cup berries of your choice (we like blueberry and raspberry)

¼ tsp powdered glucomannan (you can find this on Amazon or at your health store)

¼ tsp vanilla

Coconut oil for spraying the muffin tins

Method:

Pre-heat oven to 350 degrees

Spray your muffin tin with coconut oil

Combine everything but the berries in a mixing bowl. Whisk everything together until combined well.

Fold the berries into the batter

Spoon batter into muffin tin and bake at 350 for 20 minutes

Enjoy!

Wicked and Wilder Meat Lover's Crock Pot Chili **spicy!** (Can be modified for either plate)

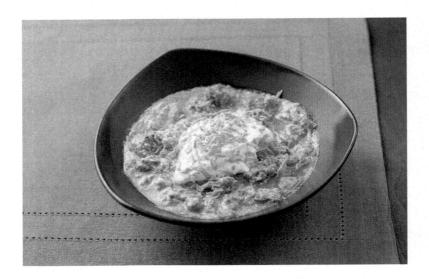

My whole family *loves* chili, especially Jack. I like to pair it with WASA crackers for my kids because they can each have their crackers the way they want; some crumble their crackers into their chili, others keep them out and spread Laughing Cow cheese on them.

We live in northern Michigan where it's -2 degrees for half the year, so we need chili to keep us warm. I usually just throw it in the crock-pot before church so we have something quick and easy when we get home. I know the chicken *and* the beef might sound weird, but just try it, you might like it!

This recipe is just right for all five of my big kids—it's not *too* spicy and it has just enough kick.

Ingredients:
1 lb boneless skinless chicken breast
2 lbs ground beef

1 small onion, diced

1 tbsp minced garlic

A bit of oil for frying

1 can lime LaCroix (tap water is also okay)

1 tsp red pepper flakes (optional)

1 can drained beans—my family likes pinto beans

2, 14oz cans of diced tomatoes—I like Rotel

1 cup plain Greek yogurt

½ block cream cheese

½ tbsp chili powder

½ tbsp cayenne

1 tbsp ground cumin

2 tsp sea salt

Juice of one lime (bottled is fine)

Method:

Pre-cook the ground beef and chicken, along with the onion, in a bit of oil. Then place in your crockpot.

Add remaining ingredients to the crockpot and mix everything together.

Turn the crockpot onto low for eight hours, or high for four hours.

Notes:

When serving add: sour cream, white cheddar cheese, and chopped cilantro.

YUM!

Perfect PB & J Smoothie
(Even the kids love it)

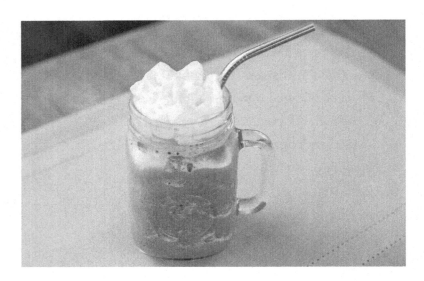

This is the perfect post-workout smoothie. It's so good we sometimes have it for dessert with just a touch of fat free Redi Whip on top. (I'm lazy, so I use the empty yogurt cup to measure).

In a blender mix together the following:

1 scoop Jay Robb Whey Isolate Strawberry protein powder

1 cup of Okios Triple Zero yogurt (Jack likes Strawberry or banana)

1 empty Triple Zero cupful frozen strawberries

1 empty Triple Zero cupful frozen blueberries

2 empty Triple Zero cupfuls unsweetened vanilla almond milk

1 small spoonful of natural peanut or almond butter

1 generous spoonful Pyure or Swerve

Pinch of sea salt

A few pieces of frozen spinach for extra protein (optional)

One scoop of collagen (optional)

Wilder Sangria

Start with your favorite dry red wine. If you don't like dry wine, just work with me here and try this anyway. All wine-lovers: TRY THIS!

1 large glass of wine
1 tsp Pyure (organic stevia sweetener)
½ cup frozen fruit or berries
A few splashes of lime juice
(mix or shake)

I know it isn't exactly real Sangria, but it will work in a pinch, and it's delicious. Once you've had one, the second one will taste even better.

Wilder Margarita

Fill a cocktail shaker with ice, and then add:
   3 oz tequila
   1 squirt lemon juice
   1 squirt lime juice
   1 packet, or to taste, True Lemon (flavored stevia)
   1 packet, or to taste, True Lime (flavored stevia)
   1 pinch salt
   (SHAKE IT UP)
   Serve with a slice of fresh lemon or lime. **#fancy**

Note:
Don't get too crazy, people. This is a family show!

French Toast Sticks
(Black Plate)

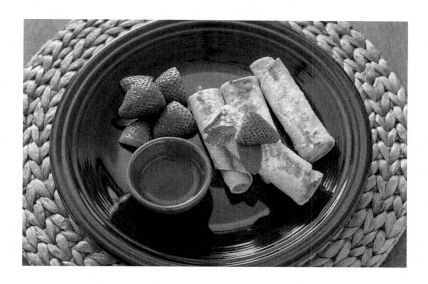

Traditional French toast was something my kids really missed, especially my littlest guys. I searched high and low until I figured out a way to make something even mom and dad could enjoy. The kids love having French Toast Sticks as a special treat on weekends,

This recipe makes 16 sticks, so big families like mine should double the recipe. These are so easy to make even the kids can help!

Ingredients:

1 package Mission low carb whole-wheat wraps (contains 8 wraps)

2 eggs

Granulated and powdered stevia

Spreadable cream cheese (1/3 fat type)

Butter for frying

1/4 cup unsweetened vanilla almond milk

Sugar free syrup (optional)

Separately mix together:
Microwave heaping three tablespoons of butter
3 tbsp granulated sugar
1 tbsp bootstrap molasses (adjust according to how much of a molasses taste you like—a little goes a long way)
1 tbsp cinnamon
Set above mixture aside.

Method:
Spread cream cheese on the inside all 8 of the wraps
Spread the molasses mixture on top of the cream cheese—I like to use a pastry brush
Roll up and cut each wrap in half to make 16 pieces.
Mix the eggs and almond milk in a wide bowl
Dip the rolled up and sliced halves into the mixture, and turn them so the eggs and milk soak in
Place 3 tbsp butter in a large pan and fry those puppies up.

Notes:
We serve them topped with the Swerve brand powdered stevia!
You can also dip them in sugar free syrup, but it isn't really needed as they're plenty sweet as is. (Our little boys love to dip them, so we go with it!)
These are the perfect morning breakfast sweet treat. I like them with a small bowl of berries. **#Fancy**

Perfect Chicken Strips
(Black Plate)

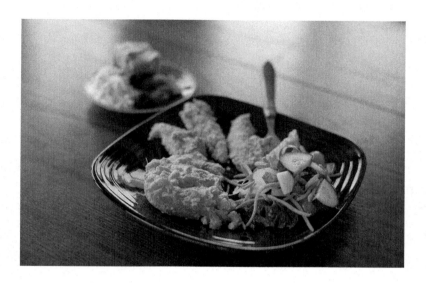

If your kids are like mine, they're going to want some good, old-fashioned chicken strips. I serve these with sweet potato fries for them and salad for mom and dad—Jack and I often just the lay the chicken strips right onto our salads. You really can't go wrong with this recipe. If you want to give them a bit of a zing, just add some cayenne.

Ingredients:

2 lbs boneless chicken, cut into strips

¾ cup almond flour

1 cup grated parmesan cheese

¼ tsp paprika

½ tsp chili powder

a dash of black pepper

1 tsp Italian herb blend

¼ teaspoon sea salt

1 tsp garlic powder

2 large eggs, stirred

½ stick butter, melted

Olive oil

Method:

Preheat oven to 400 degrees

Line a baking sheet with parchment paper.

Combine the flour, spices and cheese and place on a plate

Combine eggs and melted butter and place on a plate (a pie plate is perfect)

Dip the chicken in the eggs and butter and then roll them into the flour, spice, and cheese mixture.

Place chicken on the baking sheet and lightly drizzle with olive oil

Bake for 30-35 minutes or until golden brown.

Traverse City Cherry Lime Cheesecake

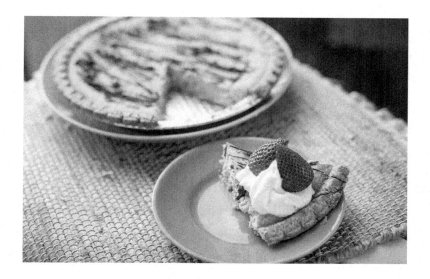

I buy premade whole-wheat crusts at my local farmer's co-op, and Whole Foods should have them, too. You can create several different flavors combos with this recipe, so experiment! We've done lemon with dark chocolate, and a peanut butter version—it depends what you're in the mood for.

Ingredients:

Filling

1/6 oz softened cream cheese

1/3 cup sour cream

½ cup heavy whipping cream (sour cream and heavy whipping cream can be substituted for each other, or use cream cheese for an even denser cake)

½ cup Swerve sweetener

1 tbsp tart cherry concentrate

2 tsp Watkins cherry extract

2 tsp vanilla extract

3 tbsp of Real Lime

pinch of salt

3 large eggs

Premade whole-wheat crust

Method:

Preheat oven to 350 degrees

Grease a springform pan with coconut oil

Place whole-wheat crust in the springform pan

Whip or mix the filling ingredients together and pour onto the piecrust.

Place the cheesecake in the preheated oven and bake for 45 – 50 minutes. It is done when the top is just slightly jiggly.

Notes:

Keep a close eye on it at the end as it can burn.

I like to drizzle some melted Lily's chocolate on top after it's cooled. My dad likes his topped with some pecans and Fat Free Reddi Whip, too. It would also be good with a side of fresh berries.

This is a special treat my family really enjoys. I hope yours does, too.

Low Carb Cheddar Biscuits
(Black Plate)

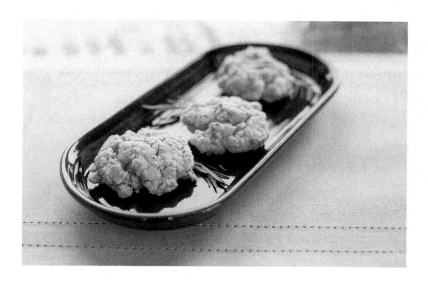

My kiddos love these family favorite biscuits. There are lots of other low carb options out there, but we really like this one that I made up. I hope you like them too!

Ingredients:
Biscuit Mix
2 cups almond flour
2 cups coconut flour
2 tbsp baking powder
4 oz shredded cheddar cheese
1 cup water
3 eggs
½ cup cream cheese (soft)
A pinch of salt
1/3 cup milk

4 tbsp butter (melted)

Method:

Preheat oven to 375 degrees

Line a baking sheet with parchment paper

In a mixing bowl combine the ingredients listed above and mix well. I like to use my big pink Kitchen Aid mixer.

Scoop the batter by the spoonful onto the baking sheet and shape into a biscuit form

Bake for 10-12 minutes.

Topping Mix

While the biscuits are baking, mix together:

1 cup melted butter

½ teaspoon salt

¼ teaspoon onion powder

¼ teaspoon dried parsley

Once the biscuits are done, brush the topping mix generously over the tops.

Enjoy!

Mom's Famous Mac & Cheese
(Black Plate)

I started making this Mac & Cheese for Easter when my firstborn was a toddler. He was obsessed with mac & cheese, and probably ate it way too much. Well…he's 12 and he's still obsessed with it; he calls this recipe my "famous" Mac and Cheese.

We only make this for special occasions—in fact, it should come with a warning label because even though the Dreamfields pasta is a great choice, the fats in this one are pretty heavy. Don't eat it too much or too often.

Ingredients:
2 boxes of Dreamfield elbow macaroni
8 tbsp butter
2 cups Half and Half
2 eggs
1, 8 oz. package of cream cheese
4 cups of your favorite cheese, shredded. (We like equal parts of Muenster, Cheddar, Monterey Jack and Colby)
S & P to taste
Cayenne pepper, garlic powder and/or dry mustard to taste

Method:
Preheat oven to 350 degrees
Coat a casserole dish with coconut oil
Cook the pasta as directed on the box, and then drain.
Combine all ingredients except the pasta in a large bowl.
Add the cooked pasta to the wet ingredients and mix well.
Pour the pasta mix into your casserole dish and place in the

oven.

Bake for about 20-25 minutes. It's done when you see it start to bubble.

Top it with a tiny bit more cheese—we REALLY like cheese—and serve with a nice green salad.

Pro Tip: make sure not to eat reheated Dreamfields if you are working on achieving your goal weight. The protective coating won't be the same once it's reheated with the result that it causes a higher insulin reaction.

Cheesy Pizza Cups
(Black Plate)

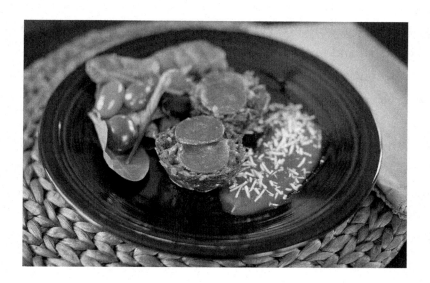

Okay, I'll admit that at one point in our lives my family was eating pizza every week. Usually on a Friday or Saturday night when I just didn't have any time to plan a meal or the energy to cook one. One of the first things my kids complained about missing, after we changed the way we ate, was pizza.

As you all know, necessity is the mother of invention. I wanted to come up with some sort of pizza my family would enjoy and something that would meet our dietary requirements. I saw something online about making cheese taco shells and this idea just came to me; I merged one of our old favorite pizza bake recipes with this, and *BAM*! Pizza magic.

The result is Cheesy Pizza Cups—they are individual pizzas made in muffin pans that kind of look like muffins, but taste like heaven.

For the crust, we often use a large Joseph's low carb flat bread, a

Mission Wrap, Ezekiel English muffins, or an egg-and-cheese pizza crust (try the Fathead low carb version—you can find the recipe online), but the version below takes the prize for my family. Yes, it takes a bit more time and prep, but the result is amazing. I serve this with a side salad and my kids gobble it right up.

Get out your muffin tin and get ready to make pizza like you've never dreamed of.

Ingredients:
(This recipe will make 8 pizza cups, but I double it for my family. Most of my family members can eat two with some sauce on the side).

Part 1:

Ingredients:
For the cheese liner shell:
One bag of grated mozzarella cheese
One bag of grated Parmesan cheese
Italian seasoning to taste

Method:
Preheat the oven to 350 degrees

Spray the muffin pan(s)—I use coconut spray, but anything will work

Next, heat up your small frying pans—I've got lots of people to cook for, so I usually do four at time.

Combine the cheeses and seasoning (only you know how much seasoning your family likes. My kids love lots of flavor, so I throw in a bunch).

Place a spoonful of the cheese and seasoning mix into a heated fry pan and fry up the cheese—It'll cook like a pancake.

Don't take your eyes off them as they can easily burn. When the edges get brown, get them into the muffin pans one at a time. Tamp them down with a spoon, so the tops come above the top of the muffin tin.

Once all eight are done, just let them sit for a few minutes and harden up.

Part 2:

Ingredients:

Combine the following:

1 lb of ground turkey, beef or even sausage, **browned** in a skillet

Minced onion to taste (optional)

1 egg

¼ tsp of pink sea salt

A bit more cheese

A tiny bit of your favorite marinara sauce—make sure the sauce is sugar-free!

Method:

Mix the filling ingredients together

Place a scoop of the mixture into each of the cheese crusts

Top each with more sauce, more mozzarella cheese, and a slice or two of pepperoni. (You can use turkey pepperoni if you prefer). **#fancy**

Bake in your preheated oven for 20 minutes!

Enjoy!

Big Bird!
(Black Plate)

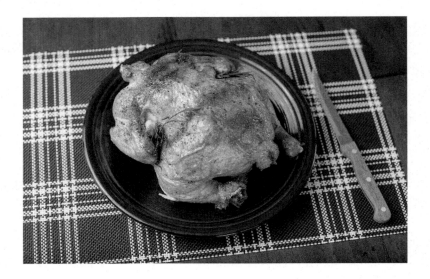

When I make roasted chicken, my kids EAT. By the time we're done with this dish, the carcass looks like velociraptors have been at it. This one is super easy to make and tastes great! Buy as many chickens as it will take to feed your family, and follow the recipe below for each one. My family can easily eat three chickens at one meal! I look for these on sale, or grab them when my farmer's co-op has some fresh ones in.

Ingredients:
Whole chicken(s)—as many as you need
Soft butter
S & P
Garlic powder
Fresh cloves of garlic, whole
An onion, quartered

Paprika

Method:

Preheat oven to 425 degrees

Rinse your chicken(s) under cold water and pat dry

Place your chicken(s) in an oven roaster; I use cast iron.

Coat the bird(s) with butter—I rub them with the stick of butter, but you can also use your hands or a fork. I don't mind getting my hands dirty, but do whatever works for you. Coconut oil is also okay here.

Sprinkle the birds with salt, pepper, garlic powder and paprika. Massage to get all the spices rubbed in.

Shove a big chunk of butter inside the bird with a few cloves of garlic and a quarter of an onion. Yes, stick it right up inside; just don't forget to wash your hands afterwards.

Roast the birds for approximately 60–75 minutes, depending on the size of the bird. Use a meat thermometer to check the internal temp of the birds: it should read at least 165 degrees before you take it out of the oven. (If you don't have a meat thermometer insert a paring knife into the thigh when you think it is done. If the juices run clear you know the bird is cooked).

Wait 10 minutes before carving and serving.

Enjoy!

Jack's Meatloaf Gone Wilder
(Gray Plate)

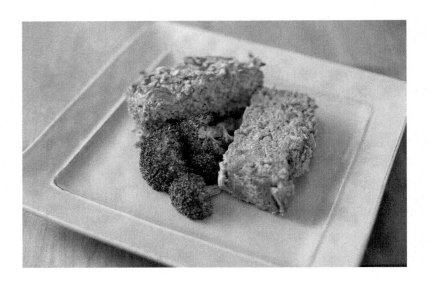

You just can't go wrong with meatloaf. I like to use ground turkey and serve the meatloaf with either some garlic green beans or mashed cauliflower on the side. And, yes, you can always use a no sugar added or reduced sugar ketchup. It tastes just as good!

Ingredients:
3lbs of ground turkey (or other ground meat)

2 bell peppers (finely chopped)

1 small onion (finely chopped)

3 tsp minced garlic

2 large eggs

1 cup grated cheddar cheese

1 tbsp cayenne pepper (depending on your preferred level of spiciness)

½ tablespoon black pepper

A few red pepper flakes (optional)

1 can tomato paste

2 tablespoons heavy cream

3 toasted and crumbled slices of Ezekiel bread

Your favorite tomato sauce

Method:

Preheat oven to 375 degrees

Mix all of the ingredients with your hands in a large bowl. I know it's gross but you'll survive.

Divide the mixture into two loaf pans.

Top with your favorite tomato sauce

You can also top it with some WASA cracker crumbles and cheese. Mmmmmm!

Bake for between 60 and 75 minutes.

Wine and Chocolate Cake
(Gray Plate)

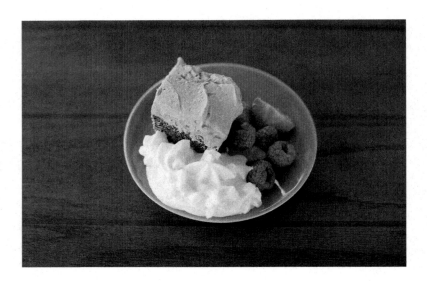

I know you might be scared to try this, but please just give it a try; it's pretty darn good. Just trust me on this. My kids eat this up and ask for more.

Cake:

Ingredients:

15 oz tin of Black Beans (drained)

6 eggs

½ cup red wine (substitute with almond milk if desired)

1 tsp vanilla

½ tsp almond extract

6 tbsp butter (melted)

½ cup cocoa powder

3 tbsp coconut flour

1 cup Swerve

1 tsp baking powder

1 tsp baking soda

½ tsp salt

Method:

Preheat oven to 350 degrees

Lightly spray a 9" square baking pan with cooking oil

Blend all wet ingredients together.

Blend all dry ingredients together.

Combine everything together and pour the batter into the pan.

Bake at 350 degrees for about 45-50 mins, or until a toothpick inserted into the center comes out clean.

Icing:

Ingredients:

1 8oz package cream cheese, softened

2 cups heavy whipping cream

3 tablespoons cocoa

4 tablespoon Swerve (confectioners style)

A pinch of salt

A dash of red wine (optional)

Method:

#WHIPITGOOD

Frost the cake when it has cooled.

Spicy Shrimp
(WHITE PLATE or BLACK PLATE)

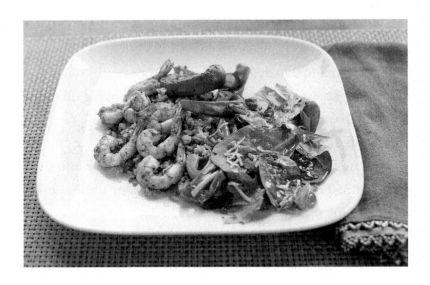

My husband isn't a huge fan of seafood, but he does like salmon and shrimp, and my second oldest son *loves* shrimp, so this is a recipe they are always asking me to make.

I get a pound or two of large, peeled, and deveined from our small town meat market. In the summer we grill it on the BBQ, in the winter we fry it up!

Ingredients:
1 or 2 lbs of large, peeled, and deveined shrimp
Chopped bell peppers, grilled
Garlic, minced if fresh, or powdered, to taste
Oil for frying (I prefer using liquid coconut oil)

Seasoning Mix: (adjust the quantities to suit your family)
Sea salt

Black pepper

Paprika

Cayenne pepper

Onion powder

Garlic powder

A pinch chili powder

Method:

Place seasoning ingredients, along with the shrimp, into a Zip-loc plastic bag and give it a good shake.

Prep the frying pan with a bit of liquid coconut oil and heat the pan

Place the grilled bell peppers and garlic in the frying pan and heat for a few minutes

Then add the bag of seasoned, uncooked shrimp to the fry pan and cook until the shrimp are nice and pink.

Notes:

Serve with a salad and a side of sprouted rice. You can also add some tomato sauce as well. You can also prepare this recipe using chicken breast instead of the shrimp

Super quick and easy!

My Kids' Favorite Veggie Dip

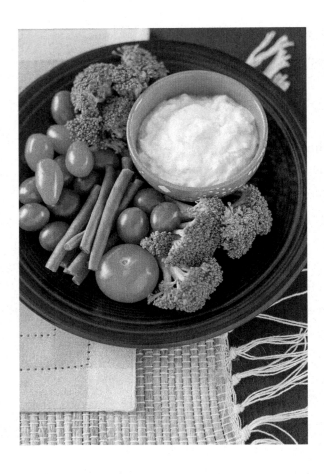

This dip is so good and so easy! I love to have it ready for my kids when they get home from school. I serve it with a big tray of bell peppers, carrots, cucumbers or whatever's in season and they dip like crazy. You can make this with your favorite cheese; we like it with cheddar or Parmesan. Making a veggie tray with this dip and keeping it in the fridge is a great way to get my kids to choose healthy veggies as a snack.

Ingredients:

1 cup sour cream (we use full fat and usually organic, depending on the price)

1 tbsp dried minced onion

1 tsp onion powder

¼ tsp garlic powder

¼ tsp salt

¼ tsp dried or fresh parsley—you can also use chives

¼ cup or more of cheese

Method:

Mix all ingredients together in one bowl and serve with veggies of your choice.

Note:

I usually double the recipe so I can keep the extra in the fridge for a few days

Enjoy!

Ru's Fruit Dip

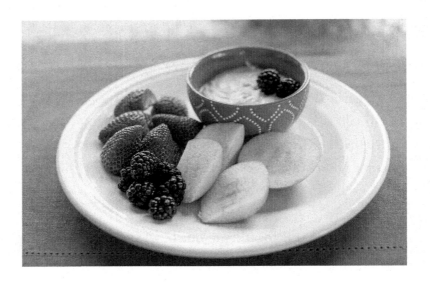

My older daughter is *obsessed* with fruit—she eats at least one apple every day. I came up with a healthy dip to replace the old one. Now she doesn't even miss the old stuff!

Ingredients:
Half a container of your favorite Triple Zero yogurt
Quarter scoop of favorite protein powder
One spoonful of peanut butter
A dash of cinnamon.
A dash of vanilla bean powder (optional)
Sliced fruit of your choice

Method:
Blend everything except the fruit. Then get dipping with the sliced fruit.

Notes:

You could also add some almond milk to the above mix for a yummy smoothie.

Don't be shy about trying different flavors and variations; Ru's favorite is strawberry yogurt and vanilla protein powder.

Mom's Fancy Spinach Omelet
(Black plate)

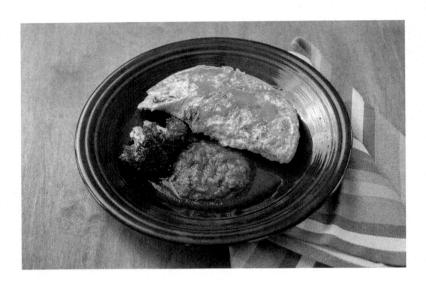

I think we've already established how much I love eggs—they are my number one superfood of choice, and I think you should eat them every day. No, your cholesterol won't go up, I promise.

Below is the recipe for the omelet I make if I have a few extra moments in the morning to get fancy. I always keep frozen spinach in my freezer because I like to sneak it into things whenever I can. It's also great with chicken, in your smoothie, with eggs, and it's *loaded* with protein. Heck, let's just add spinach to my favorite superfood list too, it's that amazing. Make one of these omelets and then try to disagree with me.

Ingredients:
Frozen spinach, or fresh. Use as much as you like.

3 eggs, well whipped. Really whip the hell out of those eggs; we want this omelet to be fluffy and perfect.

1 large spoonful of cream cheese (I usually use 1/3 fat because it's just as tasty as the regular kind.

¼ cup of salsa (I like things spicy, so I use the Field Day Organic Jalapeno Lime—you can thank me later for telling you about that stuff—but use whichever salsa you prefer).

Method:

Heat the spinach in a frying pan in a tiny bit of oil (coconut oil is best!) and some pink salt.

When the spinach is cooked, add a nice big spoonful of cream cheese and tiny bit of the salsa.

Place the whipped eggs in a separate frying pan and cook until the omelet is done on the underside.

Flip the omelet and cook the other side. Doesn't it look great?

Place the spinach mixture and the rest of the salsa in the center of the omelet—and, because I'm crazy about cheese, add even more cheddar cheese—then fold the omelet in half.

Note:

Be careful about sharing this with your kids, because they're going to want one for breakfast too, and nobody has time to make eight fancy omelets for breakfast!

Roasted Broccoli and Green Beans

Broccoli and green beans are my two favorite vegetables; if you don't eat them, you're missing out! As I've probably established by now, I like mine a bit spicy and full of flavor. If the vegetables don't have *lots* of garlic Mr. Wilder won't even touch them. I love these served with salmon. Get ready for a vegetable explosion in your mouth!

Ingredients:
Fresh broccoli florets
Green beans, trimmed
¼ cup of olive oil
Sea salt (to taste)
Red pepper flakes (to taste)
Cayenne pepper (to taste; yes, I put cayenne on everything)
2 tbsp minced garlic

Method:
Preheat oven to 375 degrees
Place the fresh broccoli and green beans on a baking sheet coated in coconut oil.

Combine remaining ingredients and brush liberally onto the veggies.

Bake for about 5 minutes, turn them over, and then cook for another 5 minutes—you can add another 5 minutes or so of cooking time if it looks like they need it.

Pro tip: You can do this with almost any veggie! Try it with some zucchini or squash too.

Loaded Baked Potato with Chicken
(White Plate)

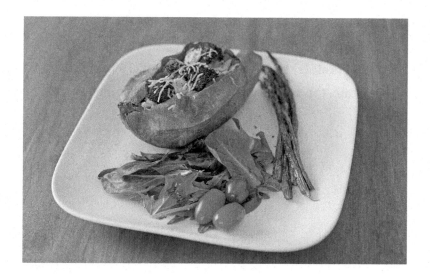

I think only the girls in my family like sweet potatoes, which is fine because it means more for us! Most people only think of loading up a regular potato, but I like to load up a sweet potato for a quick dinner—it's filling and *so* good! I serve it with a salad bar.

Ingredients:

1 large sweet potato per person

Cooked and shredded chicken

Black pepper and salt to taste

Veggies (I like broccoli and/or a tiny bit of corn—whatever you want!)

1/3 fat cream cheese, or Laughing Cow cheese

Method:

Preheat the oven to 400 degrees

Place the sweet potatoes on a baking sheet and bake at 400 degrees for about 50–60 minutes.

Once the potatoes are cooked, slice them in half; (I scoop a little out of the center to give me more room to add the fillings.

Layer on the fillings

Pop the potato(s) back in the oven for 10–15 minutes.

Once done, top with your favorite salsa, or some low-fat cheese.

Yum!

Meat Bowl is the new Taco Tuesday!
(White Plate)

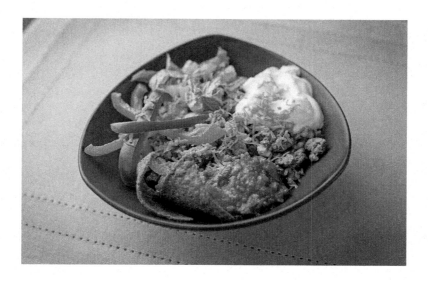

On one of our road trips, Jack and I stopped at a chain burrito place and tried to figure out the best way to eat healthy, which is how our obsession with the meat bowl was born.

We make this buffet bar style for our kids so they can choose their own veggies and other items to make it the way they like it best.

This layout is also very colorful and a great way to impress your guests. Plus, it is very simple to pull together.

Ingredients:
Lean meat such as shredded, cooked chicken
Cooked brown rice
Shredded lettuce
Salsa
Corn kernels
Sliced or diced bell peppers

Beans: kidney, pinto, chickpeas—whatever you like

Low fat sour cream

Low fat cheese, shredded

Berries of your choice

Blue corn chips

Mission low-carb, whole-wheat tortillas

Method:

Place each ingredient in a separate bowl or dish and let everyone help themselves!

Notes:

Choose lean meat; my family *loves* shredded chicken, so that's our usual. I usually offer some berries, because my kids like a tiny bit of sweet with their meals. My kids ALWAYS want some blue corn chips. If your kids really need a wrap, you can use the Mission low carb whole-wheat tortillas.

MISSION LOW CARB WRAPS

I can't say enough about these things. Mission low-carb whole-wheat wraps are the BOMB! Yes, they cost a bit more than traditional wraps, but my local store often puts them on sale and then I stock up. These things are *so* versatile and so good for you. Their texture and softness makes me prefer them over the regular wraps. We use them at nearly every meal, since they're neutral, which means you can use them on either a white or black plate.

Breakfast:

Breakfast burritos. We use bacon or sausage, cheese, and scrambled eggs in our breakfast burritos. If you want to get really fancy you can bake some cheese on top, and add some salsa. If you need a quick grab-and-go breakfast, make up a batch and freeze them for easy reheating!

Another way to serve these wraps is to coat one with cream cheese, layer on your favorite fruit and then top it with a second wrap. Lightly fry in a pan for a few minutes on each side. Our favorite filling is cream cheese and strawberry. To serve, top with powdered Swerve or sugar-free syrup, and a side of vanilla Triple Zero yogurt. It's amazing, delicious and **#fancy**.

Lunch:

Quesadillas. The kids add different meats and cheeses to their wraps, and then dip them in salsa and sour cream. So easy, quick and yummy!

Use them for any and all types of sandwiches. My little boys will even eat a PB&J on them. You can also make rollup sandwich wheels with cream cheese or Laughing Cow cheese. Just spread the wrap with the soft cheese of your choice and then roll them up like a cigar. Slice into wheels and you've got lunch!

Dinner:

We use these wraps for tacos, burritos, and enchiladas. They bake well, so you can use them in almost any dish that calls for a traditional tortilla.

You can also use them to make personal pizzas. These are super fast to make and it keeps the kids happy—they choose their own toppings, and they bake very quickly. They're surprisingly tasty. Even Mr. Wilder likes these.

WASA crackers

I've referred to these crackers many times in this book. Let me just say that the WASA cracker is an incredible thing. You've probably passed them in the grocery store without even knowing what they were. These little crackers are so versatile I've used them for breakfast, lunch, dinner, snacks, and treats! We use them so much I buy them by the case from Amazon!

WASA crackers are packed with fiber, which is vitally important for a healthy body. They have minimal carbs, and they fill you up. Whether you're craving something hearty or sweet, we can find a way to smash that craving with a WASA cracker.

Don't take my word for it, just try them!

Some of our favorite WASA cracker combinations:
- Rye WASA with natural peanut butter and all fruit jelly
- Cream cheese and all-fruit jelly and/or berries
- Any and all flavors of the Laughing Cow brand cheese with various toppings: veggies, salsa, meats
- Pizza WASA: tomato sauce, mozzarella cheese, and pepperoni (a great late night snack)
- Tomato, fresh mozzarella, and balsamic
- Sourdough WASA and your favorite cheese
- Cream cheese, nuts, and drizzled chocolate—oh yeah, I went there!

Pro tip: Throw WASA crackers into your soup and forget about croutons or other crackers. You can also crumble these into your salad for added crunch instead of using croutons.

AUTHOR NOTE

Dear Reader,

You've made it to the end of this book, and I wish I could give you a great big hug! I wrote this book for *you*. I know that for so many of us, our weight has been a life long struggle. It's personal, and often painful. It often represents a lifetime of failure, and it feels like a curse.

But things *can* be different for you.

You *can* do this! It's your time. You *WILL* succeed! You're going to KICK ASS! You have the knowledge to succeed, and I'll be right here with you every step of the way. We're going to do this together.

You ARE strong.

You ARE worthy of this positive change, and you are worthy of good health.

Don't dwell on the pain of the past; look instead toward the sweetness of the future.

Good things await you. Each new day is another chance to change the rest of your life.

Please feel free to reach out to me via social media; I would *love* to hear from you. You're in my heart and in my thoughts every day. My prayer is that women will start to make changes for their families and themselves, amazing, positive changes which will eventually end the cycle of obesity and its long list of devastating diseases.

We can do it, one mom at a time, one meal at a time.

God bless you,

Coach J

Hebrews 12:1

COOKBOOK RECOMMENDATIONS:

- *100 DAYS OF REAL FOOD* by Lisa Leake—a wonderful education about food.
- *TRIM HEALTHY MAMA* by Pearl Barrett and Serene C. Allison—my kids' favorite! These ladies are amazing at modifying family-favorite recipes. Check out THM blogger websites, too.
- *THE WHOLE 30* by Dallas Hartwig and Melissa Hartwig — perfect if you want to for start off with clean eating
- *WELL FED* by Melissa Joulwan—great ways to modify menus to include healthy Paleo options.
- *THE KETOGENIC COOKBOOK* by Jimmy Moore and Maria Emmerich—this book is just beautiful, and has some great recipes in it.
- *PRACTICAL PALEO* by Diane Sanfilippo—even though I'm not technically paleo, I love her recipes. It's a great, informative book.
- *THE PIONEER WOMAN* by Ree Drummond—I adjust these recipes to suit our needs, but they are still some of our favorites.
- *THE GRAIN BRAIN* by David Perlmutter and Kristin Loberg—fancy but solid
- *THE SEXY FOREVER RECIPE BIBLE* by Suzanne Somers—enough said.
- PINTEREST—Yes, the app. Pinterest is almost always my go-to when I want to try something new. It's an amazing resource if you want ideas or want to find a way to modify your favorite recipes. I'm sending a huge shoutout to all the bloggers who put their talents into that site for us. Some of these recipes can make a huge difference to those of us who get a hankering for something, but just can't figure out how to make it. Check Pinterest if you can't find what you're looking for in one of your cookbooks.

ADDITIONAL RESOURCES AND
READING SUGGESTIONS

Always Hungry by David Ludwig MD, Ph.D.

The Body Book by Cameron Diaz

Grain Brain by David Perlmutter MD and Kristin Loberg

Why We Get Fat and What To Do About It by Gary Taubes

Eat Fat, Lose Fat by Dr. Mary Enig and Sally Fallon

100 Days of Real Food by Lisa Leake

Choose To Lose by Chris Powell

Trim Healthy Mama Plan by Pearl Barrett and Serene Allison

Running Like A Girl: Notes on Learning to Run by Alexandra Heminsley (I *love* this book!)

Run Like A Mother by Dimity McDowell and Sarah Bowen Shea

Women's Running Magazine

www.nutritiondata.com is a great website for checking the nutritional values on your favorite whole foods.

8-WEEK CHALLENGE TESTIMONIALS

Below are testimonials from several people who've tried my plan. They inspired me and I know they will inspire you, too.

I have struggled with my weight for nearly 20 years. I was recently diagnosed with hypothyroidism and knew I was ready for a lifestyle change rather than just a new diet. I've been following Jasinda's program faithfully and have found it very easy to stick with. The first thing I noticed was I didn't miss the sugar and that I was never hungry; in fact, I ate until I was full. There was no counting calories or points, which made things stress free. Food actually tastes so much better and my energy level is through the roof! I am confident I will continue with "The Wilder Way" for many reasons. I'm no longer lethargic, and my stomach issues have disappeared. I feel good and have no problem making the best choices for my meals. I can't wait to share what I've learned with my family and friends. This experience has truly changed my life! — *Heidi M, 43*

This was the simplest change I could ever make. It was super easy to do and I really didn't have to think about it at all. All you do is eat, walk/wog, and you lose weight. It cannot be simpler than that. — *Jennifer O, 34*

I was so frustrated with my weight, so when I saw Jasinda's post asking for volunteers for a beta group for weight loss, I almost didn't care what we were going to have to do. I couldn't have imagined that eight weeks on this program would've brought so many changes. The first thing I noticed after just three days was a slight increase in energy. Nine days in and I noticed a significant decrease in heartburn. About two weeks in, I (and others) noted positive changes in my complexion (coloring and condition).

These changes have continued throughout the entire eight weeks. I've also noticed increased confidence and overall just feeling better.

One of my favorite things to come out of this experience has been that my whole family got involved. We're in the kitchen together most nights cooking dinners, and we eat out a lot less, but I love that it is not difficult at all to stay with our lifestyle changes on evenings we choose to eat out. I don't feel deprived; I can still have chocolate and ice cream. I don't have to weigh out perfect portions; I don't have to leave the table hungry or unsatisfied, no calorie counting, none of those things that made me give up on past attempts at weight loss.

I never imagined that eight weeks after starting on these changes that I would be prepping for my first 5k. The results I've achieved with minimal changes are more than I could have hoped for. I am so grateful to have been a part of this. This is not a "diet" to me. I have negative associations with that term and it sounds temporary. This is truly a lifestyle change and I have no problem staying on this track. **#WoggingWilderWay4Life** — *Andrea G, 40*

I was so excited to be chosen for this journey. The process has been empowering and easy to follow and understand. I have tried and failed many other diets before, mostly because I never really understood what to do correctly, despite reading things over and over.

With *Big Girls Do It Running*, not once have I felt hungry or deprived. I have had no cravings for any bad food. The recipes are all delicious and I love the variety. My favorite is the cheesecake. I thought I would have to just say goodbye to cheesecake in my life! I have more energy and I look forward to getting out and moving.

I take things day by day and am glad there is no true end in sight. It's the first time I am not worried about getting to the end of a diet and then messing up on the maintenance.

This is how I want to eat for the rest of my life! I have found my inner athlete. Finally, for the first time in my life, I am not defining my success as a number to reach at the end of all this. Friends and family have already noticed changes in my skin and body. Many have commented that I am happier as well. I do smile more!

The *Big Girls Do It Running* revolution has truly saved me. At the start of this year I was frustrated and didn't know where to turn or what other diet I could possibly try. I truly think Jasinda is an angel. This process is successful since she herself has experienced the struggles so many of us have. Thank you, Jasinda, for being such a light in my life. I am so grateful for you and your guidance. I feel my life is being transformed. I feel I am discovering my true self!

Thank you from the bottom of my heart! — *Donna K, 38*

This woman and her program have saved my life. A few weeks before being selected for this wonderful journey I was told I was going blind because of my diabetes. My blood sugars have always run in the 300s, even with up to six injections of insulin a day. I had given up in life.

This program has gotten me off insulin in four weeks. For the first time in 15 years my blood sugar is normal. Jasinda has helped me be able to see for many years to come. — *Sara W, 28*

I am one of the many people in this world who has tried many diets—some with great success—only to find myself eventually gaining back the weight I lost. Whether it's because I stopped counting points, or ate a bread and potato-heavy meal, one misstep would spiral out of control and the next thing I knew, all my hard work would disappear.

With the Wilder Way things have been different. For starters, the things Jasinda has asked us to cut out: sugar, bad carbs like non-sprouted bread and white potatoes, are things I don't miss. Not only do I not miss them, I feel better without them. I think that's the key to the Wilder Way success. You aren't cutting out things without a purpose or just for weight loss.

The weight loss is a pleasant side effect of your body getting the nutrition it craves. I feel better having done this plan for the past eight weeks than I have felt in years. Removing sugar from my diet has improved how I sleep and how I feel throughout the day. The food I eat tastes delicious and I enjoy eating. And because I'm eating the right thing, I get full faster and feel more satisfied longer.

If that's not enough, I'm JOGGING! Even at my lightest weight the thought of any thing close to a run would make me shudder.

As more and more people start to notice that I am looking physically better, it's hard not to want to tell them about everything I'm doing because I'm so excited about it. I truly believe this way of eating, the Wilder Way, is what is going to change my life.

As a single girl living in a big city, it's important that I am able to eat meals out, and this plan not only lets me do that, but it makes it easy to do!

The Wilder Way does take some adjustment, but once you get used to it, it feels natural and easy. It's something you can live with for the rest of your life and never feel deprived. I will always be grateful to Jasinda for inviting me to be part of this process and for helping me change my health and my body for the better. — *Michelle K, 32*

The Wilder Way has been life changing for me! It's amazing to think that eight weeks can change your life, but it completely has! Jasinda has given me the tools I need to be healthy and strong for a lifetime. Now, I can teach my children how to be healthy and strong before they become adults.

I look at things differently now, I think more about what my body needs, I read labels, and I am more knowledgeable and informed. It hasn't even been difficult; I had full faith in Jasinda, and she really came through! I was wearing a size 24 when we started this journey, and after eight weeks I have lost 18 pounds and I am now comfortably wearing a size 18! I have lost over five inches on my waist and my skin even looks healthier!

And I know this is not a temporary loss like I've had with other diets and programs, because this is NOT a diet, this is a whole new outlook on food and getting healthy. I'm getting the physical movement that my body needs, something it has not had for so long.

Thank you Jasinda for changing my life and my family's lives for the better. And I'm proud to be a part of the start of a REVOLUTION! — *Tracie W, 46*

This journey has changed my life in so many ways. The way I look at food and my body will never be the same. I've learned that I don't need a magic pill to lose weight or become healthy. Just changing the food I eat and adding FUN exercise will get me there.

I've learned that giving my body time to change is okay, and that it's okay if it doesn't happen right away. Support is number one; I wouldn't have made it this far without it. I am so grateful for this opportunity to learn a new healthy way to live my life.

My family and I are forever changed. Thank you, Jasinda, for being so unbelievably brave and for sharing your life with us. — *Chandra T, 34*

Let me start by saying that Jasinda has changed my life in so many ways! I have struggled with my weight my entire life, and I'd gotten to the point were I honestly wanted to give up. I gained 75 lbs in 2015 and was diagnosed with Polycystic Ovary Syndrome. I felt like that was the end for me. How was I ever going to defeat that? How was I going to manage losing weight with not only a broken back but with this new diagnosis?

I remember praying so hard that Jasinda would choose me when I read her post for volunteers for the beta group, but I never even dreamed I would get chosen out of the hundreds of messages she got. I cried so hard when she added me to the group, and I remember thinking, "Please God, let this be the change for me because if something doesn't give I'm not going to be around for my babies."

He answered my prayers: I truly believe Jasinda is the best thing that has happened to me in years! I went from a size 3x to a plus size XL; I was 260 pounds in December and now I'm at 238 and feel fantastic! I can exercise and not be in excruciating pain. I can eat amazing food and not feel deprived, yet I'm losing lots of inches.

I can never thank Jasinda enough for what she has done for me. Coach J, you have changed my life and I thank you from the bottom of my heart! — *Amber F, 29*

I couldn't feel more privileged to be part of this test group. The last eight weeks have taught me so many things about my body, my health, and the fact that junk is hiding in our everyday food.

I never thought I'd be able to give up sugar, soda and chips and never miss them. This isn't a diet; it's a lifestyle change that I can stick to. I'm eating well *and* losing weight! No starving. Not only am I losing in a healthy way, but also I *feel* healthier. I have energy, I'm exercising, and I'm not feeling like I'm about to quit any minute.

This program isn't hard and it's not depriving me of anything. I can have cookies and cake if I want it! They just don't have all that bad for you "death-dough" in it.

I will be forever thankful to Jasinda Wilder for inviting me on this journey to better health. I never thought I'd eat real food, not starve, *and* lose weight. I can't wait to be skinny, hot, and healthy just like Jasinda.

If I can do this, I know anyone can. — *Erecia C, 33*

When I agreed to start this program, I thought, "I cannot *wait* to change the lives of my children!" I was hopeful that I could change their eating habits and overall health. With four young children I often worry whether I am making the right decisions. Now I know for sure that I am!

My family is eating healthier and still indulging in all the things we want to eat. Jasinda has a beautiful way with words, and I have always admired her ambition and tenacity. She has truly gone above and beyond to help me, to take the time to listen to my questions and concerns, to guide my journey.

Shortly after starting this program, I realized I should be doing this program for my children. I needed to lead by example, I needed to show my family the way. And I have. I have lost weight and inches, and that makes me proud. I know this would not be possible without Jasinda's program!

The program was easy to follow, slow to start, but steady throughout. No matter what food we wanted to eat, whether it was chocolate or salad dressing, there was an alternative that was not only healthy, but it tasted good. I fully believe in the Wilder Way.

The Wilders have changed my life, changed the lives of my children, and changed my future. I am so blessed that I was chosen to help pilot this program. — *Amy B, 33*

Being 29 with PCOS has been difficult. It has been hard to find a diet and exercise program that worked. I needed to find a lifestyle change for my overall health and wellness. When Jasinda began looking for people to join her trial…I was very excited. Jasinda has inspired me for many years as an author, and now as my friend.

I trusted her with her program and she has inspired me to begin my new life. She gave me the tools to succeed with her program. My family also benefits from Jasinda's program with every meal I prepare for them. I myself am down 15 pounds and counting! I couldn't be happier with my progress. I have never felt this good and have never been happier in my life! — *Alysa D, 29*

Have you ever felt like all of the cards in the deck are stacked against you? That you feel like you don't know how much more you can take? That's where I was before this journey with *Big Girls Do It Running* began.

I had a very bad lifestyle that wasn't healthy for me, and most importantly it would end up costing me my life if I continued down that path. I was blessed enough to be selected by Jasinda for a small group to test her program before the release of this new book.

I have to say that not only am I blown away by the support I've received, but also how lucky I was to be personally coached by Jasinda. My whole outlook on food, my body, and lifestyle is completely turning around. I know changing my ways is a life-long process, but these 8 weeks have shown me I can do this for my family and myself.

Besides the weight loss, I feel like a completely different person. During my journey I experienced some life-shaking and soul-changing realizations: first, I was diagnosed with PCOS, and second, my son was going to need a very serious spinal surgery this year. I need to make myself stronger and healthier so I can face anything for him. And I will do it! **#TheWilderWay #BigGirlsDoItRunning** — *Tara R, 29*

Although I haven't lost as much weight as some of the other wonderful women in this group, I feel better than I have in a very long time. I got my ass off the couch and into the gym three days a week in spite of my hectic schedule. I have kicked my addiction to sugar, which I know now is truly evil. I never in a million years would have dreamed I would be able to do that! Diabetes runs on both sides of my family, and I'm sure I was on my way to that diagnosis…until Jasinda changed that for me.

I have learned to make the healthiest choices possible for each meal, and to plan ahead to prevent myself from failing. The dedication you have shown to me and the other women in this group is remarkable. I owe you a lot and feel a deep admiration for you. Your kindness and drive to give us the gift of health is beyond heartwarming. I love your heart, your sense of humor, your compassion, and your need to help others. I honestly don't know how you have been able to give us so much of yourself almost 24/7 for the past eight weeks.

Thank you from the bottom of my healthier heart. — *Diana K, 51*

On January 5, 2016, Jasinda Wilder asked me if I was ready to be part of The Wilder Way. Was I ready to see if eight weeks could change my life?

Eight Weeks…56 days. Could I really do this? Could I take my body, which I had been abusing for years with unhealthy habits, and completely turn things around in eight short weeks? I made a decision that day when I stepped on the scale and saw, staring back at me, a number that scared me to death; I *had* to say YES! Changes needed to happen, and *fast*. As a wife, mom, and woman I had completely lost my zest for life, as well as my confidence. It was time to put in the work and make the changes necessary for creating a healthy lifestyle for my family and me!

I knew by saying yes to The Wilder Way that I had to be 100% committed to making a huge lifestyle change. I also knew that saying no wasn't an option, this was it. If you are reading this and thinking, "Been there, done that, tried every program," believe me, I have too! And with every other thing I tried, within days, I was back to my old habits.

But, what I would come to discover is that the way Jasinda Wilder's program is laid out makes it easy for the average person to follow.

The beginning of the program made all the difference to me sticking with it. I was able to ease my body and mind into it, really taking the time to learn about food and exercise, and what they can do to fuel my body to success. Other plans I've tried in the past meant quitting cold turkey on everything, and exercising to death, which was just so hard for me to do, so I would give up! This plan had me gradually making the changes, making it much easier to keep up with.

After the first few weeks into Jasinda's program, it wasn't just the number on the scales that kept me motivated; it was the changes taking place right before my eyes that completely had me hooked on The Wilder Way lifestyle change!

Taking pictures of myself really helped me notice those everyday changes that were happening. I started to notice huge differences: my eyes were more defined, I had clearer skin, a smaller waist, no more swollen ankles, my chin and neck were shrinking, and I had a brand new energy for life! I actually *wanted* to work out, something that was completely foreign to me!

Worried about what you will eat on this plan? DON'T! Before this, my day consisted of things like frozen pizza, soda, and candy bars to get me through, but I never felt full. I cannot believe all the food I can eat in a day now. I'm eating more than I ever have before and, with Jasinda's recipes along the way, my meals are not only delicious, but nutritious, too!

If you want your life back, I urge you to try Coach J's plan. Give yourself eight weeks on The Wilder Way. It will change the way you live for the rest of your life! — *Jen G, 44*

Jasinda Wilder's plan, The Wilder Way, is educational and easy to follow. You don't have to count calories or measure out everything you eat. There are no bland, prepackaged meals, no chalky shakes to choke down, no starving yourself; you eat *REAL* food. Not only does The Wilder Way provide you with delicious new recipes to try, but also healthier versions of old favorites like cookies and cake! This is not a diet, a fad, or a gimmick, it's a plan you will want to continue for life.

I have accomplished some amazing things in just eight weeks: I've lost pounds and inches, I've gone from a sedentary lifestyle to participating in a 5K, I've kicked my pop habit (I never in my life thought I would be able to go five weeks without a soda and not miss it!). I've been able to stop taking one of my daily medications and, most importantly, I feel better physically and mentally than I have in YEARS.

I don't feel weighed down—literally and figuratively—after eating. My whole relationship with food has changed and I no longer feel guilty about eating. Not only has Jasinda changed my life, but she has given it back to me. Don't think eight weeks can change your life? Think again! — *Kerry G, 44*

I have struggled with my weight for most of my life. There have been more highs than lows, literally. I did my best on a popular, commercial weight loss regimen, losing 30 pounds in two years and three months. The trouble was I felt like I was competing, even if only with myself. If there was no change on the scale, I was a failure.

Then there was a new way, a sensible way, a Wilder Way! Nothing crazy, just smart eating, better planning, and more effective movement. I felt confident and competent; championed, and challenged.

In eight weeks, I lost 13.2 pounds, and inches off of every stubborn spot on my body. I also found a community of similar weight-worried and weary women who knew my tale all too well.

Long story short…I have pride, I have purpose, and I have power. Who would expect to gain so much from losing?

Thank you, Coach J! — *Wendy K, 48*

Eight weeks ago I pled my case to Jasinda, requesting a place in her beta test group. I had high blood pressure, skin issues, kidney issues due to weight, and overall poor health. The day I found out I was chosen, I cried. Being a single mom of two, I knew I had to give my all to this program.

Jasinda is someone I admire; and I thought if Jasinda decided that this was her calling, then I knew that this was it, my chance to take my life back. This plan is so easy. Not only for me, but my children. My daughter has severe allergies and asthma, but since making simple changes to our diets, her asthma has become virtually non-existent.

Jasinda dedicated her time, knowledge, strength, and courage to create this program, and she gave me the opportunity to take back my life, just by changing my eating—I eat real food all the time now. Then I added in running or wogging and now I can run three miles. Me! Three miles! Crazy, I know.

If you want to change your health, life, and overall outlook on your life, then join this journey. The Wilder Way is the only way.

It works, and I AM PROOF!!! — *Debbie B, 43*

Blind faith is never easy, but Jasinda's passion for not only weight loss but also life-change is infectious. Paving her own path down an already well-traveled road, Jasinda is pioneering a new lifestyle. It's more than weight loss. More than a lifestyle change. Jasinda's plan may very well be your last stop on the weight loss roller coaster.

We own our weight. The world may have you thinking differently, but your weight and the reason(s) you hold on to it is personal. Whatever your struggle may be, Jasinda's plan will have you reevaluating everything you think you know about weight loss. Week by week you will learn that you're strong enough. That you have the determination. That you're worth it.

Why buy a book about a topic that has been worked and reworked? Well, actions speak louder than words. Jasinda has proven this process works. She is talking the talk and walking the walk. She is a talented author who has documented her personal journey and has chosen to share that journey with the world. Her hope is to better the life of at least one person, but I feel she will help change the world.

Am I a believer? Well, 40 pounds down, my migraines are at a minimum, my skin looks great, I have tons of energy, and no more airplane seatbelt extensions! Is this a quick fix? No. I didn't put this weight on overnight, and I won't lose it overnight. It's a lifestyle, not a diet. A way of life that not only betters me, but the people around me. I am a work in process. I will never give up on myself. Even when I was at my heaviest there was always a part of me that kept trying, in some way.

You have nothing to lose but weight, right? What better way to learn than with someone who has been in the trenches, put in the work, done the research, and has found a solution that works? I believe in Jasinda as a friend, an author, and now as a pioneer. You will too! — *Pamela C, 37*

Upon joining *Big Girls Do It Running*, I was depressed, unmotivated, and complacent. When I thought about going to the gym, or starting a new diet, I always told myself, "there is always tomorrow," but tomorrow always came and went, and led to constant excuses and giving up. I was torn between wanting to be healthy but feeling like I didn't know where to begin.

Then I was chosen to be in this revolution, and little did I know it would be life changing! It sparked a motivation in me. For once in my life I had an "I *can* do it" attitude! I felt stronger, energized, healthier, and more alive.

Jasinda introduced us to wogging and, at first, I got scared and didn't think I could hit the pavement, and that my body wasn't made to run. Little did I know the opposite was true, and I pushed myself to see if I could go farther, faster and to see if I could run without stopping to catch my breath.

With this program, I have achieved more in eight weeks than with any other program I've tried. I also feel the best I have in my entire life! My relationship with food and my body has changed, which I never thought was possible…and it was all due to Jasinda's constant support, and her program. — *Kelly L, 28*

Thank you, Jasinda Wilder, for deciding to share what you learned with other women, thank you for picking me to join this amazing group of women who were all ready to change their lives.

I have been talking for the last few years about losing weight, but it never happened. I was determined this year that I was going to make it happen, and then you, Jasinda, appeared!

My mom died of breast cancer at age 46. I just turned 44. The closer I get to 46, the more fearful I become. I have so much life to live and so many things I want to do. While I can't prevent breast cancer, I can do something about heart disease, diabetes, and other health issues I'm at risk of because of my genetics.

This plan has given me the strength to fight hard for my body and my life. I now know I can do this! Are there days when I want to throw in the towel and give up? Yep! But I see the bigger picture, and I pull up my big girl panties and I keep going, because I'm down 11 pounds and I can see it working.

I look at all the other ladies in this group, and I'm motivated. Thank you all so much for helping me get back to the me that's not ashamed of looking in the mirror. The me that isn't ashamed to take pictures. I didn't really take a full body picture in the beginning because I was ashamed and embarrassed of what I had let happen to my body. I'm working my way back to me, and I'm so very thankful to you, Jasinda. I'm still scared some days that I'm messing up, but I won't quit! — *Camisha C, 44*

This 8-week program has educated me more than anything else I have tried. There are so many lies in the food industry and, sadly, most companies don't care about our health. Jasinda's book has educated me on how to read labels and what to look for. Before taking part in this trial, knowing what to eat was very confusing. But having her support and motivation through these eight weeks has been like nothing else. She is hardcore, but in a fun way!

Thank you for teaching me about health and about myself, Jasinda, and thank you to all the other ladies in this 8-week group. We rocked it! — *Ashlee B, 31*

I have not battled with obesity my whole life; in fact, I was the quintessential skinny girl growing up. "Bean Pole and Olive Oil" is what they used to call me. I could pretty much eat anything I wanted.

The battle started when I got to college. You know the "Freshman Fifteen" everyone talks about? Yeah, mine was more like the "Freshman Fifty." I was working at McDonald's and I thought I could eat anything I wanted and not gain a pound. I was wrong—I gained *lots* of weight. I eventually drifted to my second fast food job, Hardee's. I continued the same terrible eating habits and eventually ballooned to around 350 lbs. I was shocked because I weighed 195 lbs in high school.

At first you don't think about how much of an impact weight has on your body, but eventually many ailments came with the excess weight I was carrying. I developed varicose veins in both legs and when I had my first child, I developed preeclampsia and the fear of diabetes.

I almost lost my child and my life because my weight was out of control. Thankfully, however, both of us survived and I vowed to be healthier. Well, that didn't last too long, and before you know it I was having my second child and I still had the same health issues; this time my leg had swollen to twice its normal size. I was confined to bed because they feared I had a blood clot and they didn't want it to travel. I had a healthy baby, but momma wasn't healthy.

I struggled with my weight fluctuating for years. I've tried Weight Watchers, diet pills, and many other programs that were quick fixes but weren't long term. Each time I gained the weight back fast, plus more.

When Jasinda posted that she was looking for women to join her *Big Girls Do It Running* group, I said to myself, "What the hell, I've tried everything, so why not try this too?"

I was skeptical when I started this journey. Jasinda's advice and support is truly valuable. She and the amazing group of women in the group helped me celebrate my successes, and kept me focused on my goal. Jasinda didn't let me beat myself up when I had a slip up, and she helped me remember how far I had come at each step of the journey. Her loving words are what kept me going. "Focus on the next meal," she would say.

Her plan didn't have me completely cutting out everything I loved; instead it had me finding healthier, alternative choices. I was excited about what I got to eat, and I didn't feel deprived because of what I couldn't eat. She challenged me to slowly introduce exercise and eventually she had me wogging two miles! I found myself accomplishing things I'd never done before.

This entire process made me realize that weight loss is not a quick fix. No, *wham, bam, thank you ma'am*. It takes time—it is a complete life change, a happy shock to your heart, body and mind. I now have more confidence than I've had in years, and I finally feel comfortable in my clothes.

I'm still learning, growing, succeeding, and failing. And that's okay because I know there is an amazing group of woman there to support me along the way. I am completely grateful for Jasinda's passion to help others lead healthy lives. Thank you. I will forever be indebted to you. — *Monique W, 30*

Beta Test Group Results:

Upon completion of the 8-Week trial, members of the group experienced the following:

- Normal blood sugars
- Improved skin condition
- Improved sleep
- Increased energy
- Increased libido
- Improvement with anxiety and depression
- Improvement with lethargy
- Total weight loss of 365 pounds and 130 inches around the waist, across 25 participants from all ages, races, and socio-economic backgrounds.

"God meant for my body to be healthy and strong.
I am worth the time it will take to make myself stronger and healthier.

It won't be easy, *but it will be worth it.*
Yes, it's okay to do this for those who love me as well, but this is for me.
I was beautiful then, I am beautiful now, and I will be beautiful tomorrow.

I CAN DO THIS.

I can do this despite feeling like I can't, or that I've been told I can't.
My body is beautiful at any size.
My body is going to be unstoppable when I'm healthier and stronger, so watch out!
NOTHING WILL DEFINE ME.

Nothing will stop me.
I CAN DO THIS!"

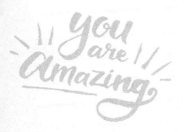

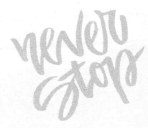

Grocery List

Oikos Triple 0 yogurt

Ezekiel brand breads & cereals – they even have English muffins

WASA brand crackers

Berries

Eggs – farm fresh are the best!

Applegate brand sausages (OMG, so good!)

Pancakes made from oats

Veggies – eat them in season to save. Local farmer's markets are the awesome.

Lily's brand chocolate

Dreamfields brand pasta

Meat & seafood – we try to do local, lean and grass fed. Laura's beef is a great brand

Almond milk – we love Califia Farms brand

Fairlife brand milk

Breyer's Carb Smart ice cream

Nuts – my family loves nuts, especially almonds and cashews

Baked blue corn chips

Mission brand low carb wraps (we use these for roll ups in place of sandwiches and for taco Tuesday)

Kerry's Gold brand butter

Sour cream – yep, the real stuff

Cheese – the real stuff, but nothing processed

Oils – I use mostly coconut and olive oil

Lots of herbs and spices. Don't think your kids won't like them, mine want everything seasoned now.

Quest brand protein bars – great after a run or workout

Lesser Evil brand popcorn – found on Amazon

Bai 5 brand drinks

Vitamin Water Zero

Grocery List

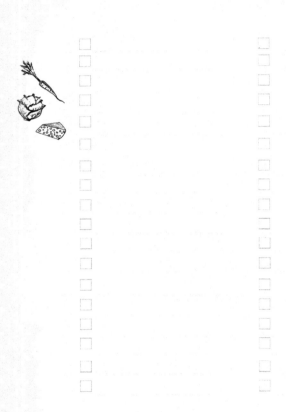

Weekly Meal Planner

	breakfast	lunch	snack	dinner
SUNDAY	☐ white plate ☐ black plate	☐ white plate ☐ black plate	☐ white plate ☐ black plate	☐ white plate ☐ black plate
MONDAY	☐ white plate ☐ black plate	☐ white plate ☐ black plate	☐ white plate ☐ black plate	☐ white plate ☐ black plate
TUESDAY	☐ white plate ☐ black plate	☐ white plate ☐ black plate	☐ white plate ☐ black plate	☐ white plate ☐ black plate
WEDNESDAY	☐ white plate ☐ black plate	☐ white plate ☐ black plate	☐ white plate ☐ black plate	☐ white plate ☐ black plate
THURSDAY	☐ white plate ☐ black plate	☐ white plate ☐ black plate	☐ white plate ☐ black plate	☐ white plate ☐ black plate
FRIDAY	☐ white plate ☐ black plate	☐ white plate ☐ black plate	☐ white plate ☐ black plate	☐ white plate ☐ black plate
SATURDAY	☐ white plate ☐ black plate	☐ white plate ☐ black plate	☐ white plate ☐ black plate	☐ white plate ☐ black plate

The three possible plates for your meal

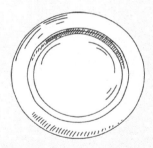

THE BLACK PLATE
Protein + Fat(s)

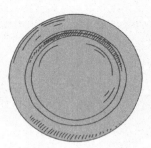

THE WHITE PLATE
Protein + Carbohydrates and starches

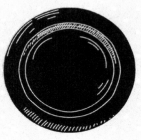

THE GRAY PLATE
Protein + Fat(s) + Carbohydrates/starches
(4-5 of these per week max)

FATS

nuts and nut butters
avocado
butter
cheese
cream
mayo
oils
whole eggs
full fat meats
chocolate
ice cream *
nut flour

*Bryers Carb Smart
and no sugar added coconut dream

Neutral Choices

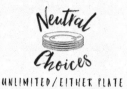

UNLIMITED/EITHER PLATE

spices
lemons & limes
berries
asparagus
broccoli
cabbage
cauliflower
celery
cucumber
egg plant
green beans
all greens
mushrooms
onions
peppers
sprouts
squash
tomatoes (salsa)
zucchini
Dreamfields pasta
Okios 000 yogurt
Low carb/Whole wheat
Mission wraps

CARBS/STARCHES

sprouted breads
sprouted cereal
blue corn chips
old fashioned oats
apples
apricots
bananas
grapes
kiwi
melon
oranges/tangerines
peaches
nectarines
pears
pineapple
plums
popcorn
quinoa
rice (brown, wild)
beans
hummus
lentils
carrots
corn
potatoes (sweet)
WASA crackers (4)

Measurements

	arms	chest	waist	hips	thighs	" lost
JAN						
FEB						
MAR						
APR						
MAY						
JUNE						
JULY						
AUG						
SEPT						
OCT						
NOV						
DEC						
total lost						

You are doing fantastic!

How I'm feeling

date:

place photo here

Hello
beautiful!

Running Log

date	Time	distance	walking speed	running speed	notes

get out and wog!

Journal

Think Positive

I CAN DO THIS!

For printable versions of the worksheets: please visit,
www.biggirlsdoitrunning.com.

RECIPE INDEX

CPSIA information can be obtained
at www.ICGtesting.com
Printed in the USA
LVOW01*1623270716

498003LV00013B/156/P